## TOTAL NUTRITION, TOTAL HEALTH

There are 22 basic elements in the human body—
enzymes, hormones, vitamins, amino acids and
others—which must be renewed by nutrient intake. No one food contains all of them . . .

. . . except bee pollen.

The healing, rejuvenating, and disease-fighting
effects of this total nutrient are hard to believe,
yet are fully documented. Aging, digestive upsets,
prostate diseases, sore throats, acne, fatigue,
sexual problems, allergies, and a host of other
conditions have been successfully treated by the
use of bee pollen—and the vigorous good health
maintained by whole populations who make it a
staple of their diets is equally well attested.

Carlson Wade presents the facts about bee pollen, gathered from around the world, in this fas-
cinating study of the nature and workings of the
"all-purpose" food—

THE ESSENCE OF LIFE ITSELF

*Also by Carlson Wade*

Vitamins and Other Food Supplements
Fats, Oils and Cholesterol
Hypertension and Your Diet
Arthritis, Nutrition and Natural Therapy
Water and Your Health (with Allen E. Banik, O.D.)

# Carlson Wade's
## NEW FACT/BOOK ON

# Bee Pollen and Your Health

Keats Publishing, Inc.          New Canaan, Connecticut

*To the pollen-making bee . . . foundation of life!*

# TABLE OF CONTENTS

*Bee Pollen*
*and*
*Your Health*

# INTRODUCTION

AS A FOOD, bee pollen may well be considered older than mankind. Bees reportedly buzzed over our planet long before humans walked in the woods and forests. The foods made by bees in the form of honey and pollen have long sustained animals and people. These foods can provide complete nourishment to maintain life for an extended period of time, even without the ordinary forms of essential nutrients.

In the past decade, science has discovered that bee pollen—the male sperm cells of flowering plants—contains a miracle concentration of nearly all the known nutrients.

Bee pollen is considered a potent healer, a source of regenerative power which can pervade the body. It is said to have been the secret "ambrosia" eaten by the ancient gods to acquire eternal youth. Today, scientists realize that bee pollen does contain healing properties that create a feeling of rejuvenation within the body. New scientific discoveries reveal how it has been able to extend the life span as well as heal ailments.

Bee pollen is a timeless wonder food, an all-natural creation, even a source of life.

Man's search for youth leads to the beehive. This book takes you on the journey to the ambrosia of the gods in the eternal quest for youth.

# CHAPTER 1

## MAN'S SEARCH FOR YOUTH FROM THE BEEHIVE

Plant pollen, a substance carried by bees back to their hives to be stored as food, has long been considered a source of youth and vitality for mankind. Bee pollen, as it is called today, as well as honey, have been mentioned in ancient writings since the beginnings of time. The Talmud, the Bible, the Koran (the Code of Islam), along with the scrolls of the Orient, ancient Greece, Rome, the countries of the Middle East as well as those of Russia and the Slavic regions all praise bee pollen and honey as a source of perpetual youth and health for mankind. They are natural foods, containing a high concentrate of nearly all known nutrients that do more than just nourish the body. They create a form of internal revitalization, a feeling of youthful energy. Because of this healing power, bee pollen and honey have long fascinated scientists, researchers and those who search for a natural way to body and mind rejuvenation. Bee pollen may well be considered the world's first health food.

The history of mankind parallels the history of the pollen-carrying bees. In prehistoric and primitive times, as man wandered the four corners of the world the bees went along with his cattle, sheep, horses and seeds for planting. Wherever man settled, even for a short time, to cultivate land, to till soil, to fish the streams, a colony of bees would accompany the pioneers, build a hive and start to make honey with the use of pollen. When people moved on, some of the bees would go along to prepare new hives in the next settlement. These hives would provide sources of honey and pollen to be used for sustenance by the settlers. Often, they served as the total source of nourishment—and healing of illness—for the settlers. The bee may well be considered mankind's best friend.

Long before the invention of parchment or paper, the ancients were inscribing their praise of bees, pollen and honey. The ancient peoples of Egypt, India and Peru made petroglyphs (carvings) of these winged insects and the products they created. In ancient Egypt, land of the Pharaohs, temples, obelisks and sarcophagi extolled the virtue of bees. The Flamic and Pamphilic obelisks on the famous Rosetta stone, the pillars of the Temple of Karnak all contain inscriptions about the value of the bees. Bee designs appear on the sarcophagus of Rameses III (Twentieth Dynasty, 1198-1167 B.C.). King Menes, founder of the First Dynasty of Egyptian kings, was known as "Royal Keeper of Bees" during his reign, believed to be about 3400 B.C. Wall paintings in the royal tombs represent the bee and its products. Nearly all funeral vaults pictorially represented the bee, honey and the honeycomb as well as bee pollen. The entire wall of the tomb of Pa-Ba-Sa, believed to have reigned around 4000 B.C., is decorated with rows of bees. Murals in many tombs also depicted all phases of the honey gathering, the accumulating of pollen and the worship of the bee as the source of eternal life.

The Egyptian papyri, discussing the older civilization in the world, contain many references to honey and its healing values. Bee pollen is also described as "life-giving dust," and instructions are given for offering both honey and pollen to the deities.

The ancient Egyptians worshiped the bees because they are the only creatures which are entirely subservient to a leader. When Egyptian kings would sign a paper, they would make a bee inscription beside it to symbolize their power over all others.

In India, a religious writing known as the *Rig-Veda*, written about 1500 B.C., contains many references to honey. A devout Hindu would turn his right side toward a beehive as if he were passing a deity. Krishna, the Hindu deity, was always symbolized by a bee. He was called *madhava* or "born in honey," and his image was sprinkled with pollen. The Hindus believed that the eating of honey and pollen would create good health as well as happiness and wisdom.

During religious ceremonies, the Hindus drink a combination of honey, pollen and curds known as *madhuparka*. They toast all others, as well as their deities, with this mixture and consider it an exhilarating tonic.

The followers of Mohammed, the founder of Islam, cannot partake of fermented alcoholic beverages; they were directed instead to drink water with honey. When Mohammed journeyed forth to the seventh heaven, he faced Christ, who directed the Archangel Gabriel to offer him a cup filled with honey. The Mohammedans believe Paradise to be a land in which "rivers flow with honey" and the countryside is abundant with gardens and pollen.

In the Orient, honey and pollen were used both for medicinal purposes and as an adjunct to regular diets. Often, a mixture of honey and pollen was used as a poultice on wounds. It was also used in combination with fruit or vegetable juices as a health tonic.

Throughout the writings of ancient Greece, honey and pollen appear to be vital factors. Homer's *Iliad* contains many references to "the food of kings." Athenians used honey and pollen almost daily, gathered from hives around Mount Hymettus. This particular mountain, southeast of Athens, was covered with fragrant wild blossoms such as thyme and the air was radiant with the perfume of these blooms. Bees gathered pollen from the thyme to make a fragrant honey. Grecians would then scoop up both pollen and the honey, which they claimed gave them vigor, strength and youthfulness.

Attica, the ancient Greek city in the eastern region, was said to have some twenty thousand hives within its forty square miles during the reign of Pericles (429 B.C.). It is said that people came from a great distance to benefit from honey and pollen, to improve their health and help them recover from their ailments.

Honey and pollen were also in general use during the Roman Empire. Honey farms proliferated throughout the entire Mediterranean region. Apiculture (beekeeping) flourished during the Second Punic War (218-201 B.C.). The Romans made Virgil their official poet laureate of bees. His *Aeneid* praised honey and pollen as "sweet-scented, fragrant with thyme."

Pliny, in the eleventh book of his *Natural History* (about A.D. 50) devoted a number of chapters to pollen "which the bees collect from the sweet juices of flowers, so beneficial to health."

Nearly all the Latin writers praised honey. Cicero (106-43 B.C.) in *De Senectute* pointed to its virtues, the way it can promote strength and long life.

When a guest came into a Roman home, he was welcomed with this greeting: "Here is honey and pollen, provided by the gods, to protect your health."

Long before the Romans conquered what is today known as Great Britain, the inhabitants of the British Isles considered honey and pollen as part of their staple diet. An historian, Tickner Edwardes, writing in *The Lore of the Honey Bee*, a number of decades ago, tells that ". . . among the Anglo-Saxons, the beehives supplied and nourished the entire nation, from the king down to the poorest serf, with more than just food but with drink, as well. Britain was known among the early Druid writers as the Isle of Honey."

Edwardes then says, "British history begins with the record of the first voyage of the Phoenicians, who adventuring farther than any of their intrepid race, chanced upon the Scilly Isles and the neighboring coast of Cornwall and thence brought back their first cargo of tin.

"The whereabouts of the Phoenician 'country of tin' remained a secret probably for ages, jealously guarded by these ancient mariners, the first true seamen that the world had ever known. It is known that little tin containers filled with honey and pollen were on the ships of these ancient voyagers and served to sustain them during their travels."

Welsh and Celtic legends are abundant with references to honey and pollen as well as to sparkling mead and other honey beverages. (Mead was made of four-fifths wine, one-fifth honey and a tablespoon of pollen. Warmed, then cooled, it was regarded as a life-giving beverage.)

Tributes and taxes were exacted in terms of honey and pollen, as well as mead. Chieftains of the tribes in ancient Britain would demand certain portions of honey and pollen from subjects, depending upon their earnings.

Many ancient writings also refer to the use of honey and pollen for cooking. Nearly all types of meat and fish dishes, stews, soups, even salads and porridge contained honey and pollen in one form or another. Many of the sweets for which England came to be known so well were largely sweetened with honey and pollen, while sugar was considered less stimulating!

Most of the people of early England used honey, together with ale or other alcoholic beverages. Nearly all inns had a sign of the alewife, a stout and buxom woman who held two cups in her hands, symbolizing honey and pollen that would be combined and then made into a liquor.

German apiculture was far advanced, prior to the Roman invasion. Fragments of the writings of Pytheas, contemporary of Alexander the Great (356-323 B.C.), tell of his journeys of exploration. He found that *meth* (a form of honey wine referred to in the Nibelungen Saga) was used in ancient Alamannia and that everyone ate thick chunks of black bread covered with honey and sprinkled with pollen. It is also said that enormous honeycombs could be found in almost all hollow tree trunks.

Charlemagne, emperor of the West (who ruled A.D. 800-814), wrote in his *Capitulares Karlomanni* that the people of the region used honey and pollen almost daily. Furthermore, the people were required by law to prepare a total accounting or inventory yearly of their supply of honey and pollen. The great monasteries that flourished throughout this era also cultivated bees and gathered honey and pollen. Farmers and residents had to pay taxes in the form of honey, wax and jars of pollen. Many honey festivals were held throughout the region. It was considered a gesture of good faith to give a little gift of honey or pollen to someone else.

The French, too, revered honey and pollen. Beekeepers and anyone who gathered honey and pollen in the open forests and woods had to pay heavy taxes in the form of their products.

Throughout the Slavic region, beehives proliferated. Herodotus (fifth century B.C. Greek historian) says that at certain intersections the bees were so thick it was impossible to go across the river. When the Turks wanted to fight back enemy crossings at the Danube, they would hurl buzzing beehives that would terrify the hostile invaders. Hungary was also known as a center of beekeeping. Taxes were paid in honey and pollen. All the other Slavic peoples loved honey and pollen; they used them on thick chunks of black bread, and also in beverages.

In the United States, pioneers came to an established worship of the bee. The Mexicans, drawing from their rich Aztec and Mayan heritage, worshiped the bee and collected honey and pollen for offering to their deities as well as for their own use. Hieroglyphic carvings are replete with symbols of bees, honeycombs and pollen, as well as the human figure bearing heavy jugs of honey to be offered as a tribute to a deity or a ruler or both.

Early Americans encountered bees, hives, honey and pollen from the start. With lavish forests, vegetation, thick woods and lush acres of flowers, bees proliferated, and honey as well as pollen could be had for the gathering. Honey production increased rapidly from the early days of the colonists; there is hardly a city today in the United States that does not have available a supply of honey and pollen for table use.

### The Healing Properties of Honey and Pollen

The use of honey for healing has long been known. In the Bible, Solomon says (Proverbs 24:13), "My son, eat thou honey, for it is good." It is said that honey with pollen could make one healthy as well as youthful in body and mind. Moses, when left in the fields, would use honey and pollen for nourishment. Jonathan, the son of Saul, ate honey and pollen and was said to have enjoyed better vision. It is also written that Jonathan was making a journey through a thick woodsy area while battling the Philistines. He had been wounded and was at the point of exhaustion. He came upon a beehive which dripped honey. He ate some of the honey, then scooped out some pollen found on the bottom of the beehive. Almost at once, his strength was restored and his vigor doubled.

Saint Ambrose (bishop of Milan, approximately A.D. 340-397) said in his writings, "The fruit of the Bees is desired of all, and is equally sweet to Kings and Beggars and it is not only pleasing but profitable and healthful, it sweetens their mouths, cures their wounds and conveys remedies to inward ulcers."

In the sixteenth chapter of the Koran, a section entitled "The Bee" says, "There proceedeth from their bellies a liquor of various colour, wherein is medicine for men." (The various colors refers to many shades of honey, depending upon its source.) Mohammed also declared, "Honey is a remedy for all diseases." He directed that honey be eaten not only because it was a tasty food but also because it had healing properties and could create good fortune.

Hippocrates, considered the father of modern medicine, wrote, "Honey and pollen cause warmth, clean sores and ulcers, soften hard ulcers of the lips, heal carbuncles and running sores."

In the days before chemicalized medicine, honey and pollen were used for healing. Here are some of the folk remedies from past and present times:

**Disinfectant.** Take several tablespoons of honey and pollen daily for internal disinfection. These foods are high in potassium, which creates a hygroscopic power (the ability to draw off moisture). Because germs thrive in moisture, this effect will deprive them of their nourishment and they die, therefore disinfecting your body.

**Magic Healer.** Egyptians applied honey to open wounds, and watched the healing take place. Orientals applied an ointment of honey and pollen to open scabs or skin breakouts to promote healing. The ancient Hebrew physicians combined honey with pollen for a dressing atop ulcerated wounds, burns and boils.

**Folk Healing with Honey and Pollen.** South American Indians used honey and pollen as a dressing for open wounds. Farm people of the Slavic region combine honey, pollen and flour to use as a natural ointment upon wounds and burns. Norse explorers used a sprinkling of pollen on burns and wounds to heal them. In modern times, Scandinavian people combine honey, pollen and cod liver oil to use as an ointment on wounds or blemishes for natural healing.

**Respiratory Ailments.** In many regions of Europe, farm people use a combination of honey and pollen to help heal respiratory ailments. It is sipped slowly from a spoon to soothe the itching throat. It is also believed to heal bronchial disorders as well as allergies such as asthma, and a honey-pollen poultice is often applied around the throat. A few drops of slightly warmed honey pollen in the ears eases pain, ringing or inflammation.

**Honey + Pollen + Warm Milk = Healthy Throat.**

Many opera singers add some honey and pollen to a glass of warm milk and sip slowly. This helps soothe the throat and promote golden tones.

**Respiratory Relief.** Folklorists suggest that you dissolve 1 tablespoon of honey, 1 teaspoon bee pollen and some lemon juice in a cup of freshly boiled water. Stir vigorously until dissolved. Sip slowly. This mixture, they say, soothes the respiratory distress, sore throat and other symptoms of lung discomfort.

**Natural Sleeping Tonic.** Early New England settlers prepared this mixture: combine 4 tablespoons honey, 2 teaspoons pollen, 3 teaspoons apple cider vinegar in a cup of freshly boiled water. Sip slowly. Taken especially at bedtime, it is said to be a marvelous and all-natural sleeping tonic.

**Oriental Youth Elixir.** Combine 2 tablespoons honey, 2 teaspoons pollen, ½ teaspoon chopped ginseng herb and dried orange peel. Take with a spoon. Oriental healers believe that this creates a feeling of total rejuvenation and vitality.

**Natural Regulatory Reaction.** You can use honey and pollen to help solve problems of irregularity. When you take honey with pollen, either in liquids or as a topping on thick black bread, your metabolic system becomes stabilized, relieving constipation or diarrhea.

**Basic Digestive Aid.** Honey and pollen do not ferment in the digestive system because they are inverted sugars. They are easily absorbed and do not attract bacteria. Furthermore, the flavor of these foods seems to perk up the appetite and helps to create a healthy desire for nourishing food. Honey with pollen creates a lubricating effect. The fatty acid content will improve peristalsis so that there is a normalizing of the digestive system, creating healthy regularity.

**Creates Muscular Vigor.** The billions of cells and tissues in your muscles require sugar for energy. When muscles are active, they use up nearly four times as much glycogen as when at rest. It is a biological-scientific discovery that predigested sugars in bee pollen convert rapidly in the bloodstream to glycogen. Almost immediately after taking it there is a speedy natural carbohydrate assimilation, and nourishment is sent to your muscle cells and tissues, resulting in a feeling of energy and vigor.

**Kidney-Bladder Revitalization.** Take honey with pollen by the spoonful or mixed in with a liquid for a natural diuretic action. In conditions of pyelitis (inflammation of the kidney), honey helps hasten the release of urine, thereby cleansing both the kidneys and the bladder and creating a beneficial antiseptic reaction.

**Sore Throat.** Many professional speakers and singers use honey and pollen to clear away obstructions in the throat. A popular throat-pleaser is prepared by mixing 3 parts honey with 1 part pollen and 1 part compound tincture of benzoin (available at herbal pharmacies). Take by the teaspoon. It feels smooth as it goes down the throat, sweeping away so-called cobwebs.

**Soothing Gargle.** Folklorists suggest adding 1 tablespoon pollen, 3½ ounces honey and 1 ounce alum (from herbal pharmacy) to 1 quart water. Stir until blended. Then gargle with this mixture throughout the day. Very soothing for itchy, scratchy throats.

From the earliest days, man has searched for a substance that will help perpetuate the feeling of youth. His search has almost always led him to the beehive and products made by these winged creatures who appear to predate man and other living beings. Bees appear to have a built-in eternal survival power that has made them nature's oldest surviving creatures. The secret for their stamina may well be in the hive . . . in the form of honey but even more in the form of pollen.

# CHAPTER 2

## BEE POLLEN: LATEST SCIENTIFIC DISCOVERY

Bee pollen is one of the world's oldest youth foods. It is now being recognized by scientists throughout the world as a substance that can help promote youthful feeling, build resistance to ailments, help boost healing powers and provide dynamic energy. The scientific discovery of the youth-building powers of bee pollen in the current century was made some three decades ago by Russian biologist and experimental botanist, Nicolai Tsitsin, as reported in the *London Sunday Express* (April 15, 1945):

"There are more than 200 people living in the Soviet Union who claim to be over 100 years old. We sent out letters to them to answer three questions: What was their age, how had they earned a living most of their lives, and what had been their principal food. We got 150 replies out of the 200 letters.

"We made a very interesting discovery. The answers showed that a large number of them were beekeepers. But all of them, without exception, said that their principal food always had been honey.

"We found out that in each," continues Dr. Tsitsin of the Longevity Institute of the USSR, "it wasn't really honey these people ate, *but the waste matter in the bottom of the beehive.* They were poor and they sold all the pure honey in the market and kept only the residue for themselves." Dr. Tsitsin explains that biologists studied this residue and discovered that a large part of this honey scrap was not honey at all—but almost pure pollen, which falls off the bees' legs while they deposit their honey.

Dr. Tsitsin felt that longevity factors in this bee pollen were able to give the beekeepers their robust health, even at the age of a hundred.

Bee pollen is the ultrafine powder that makes up the male element of a flower. Bees gather this pollen in microscopic amounts and bring it into the hive for food. By instinct and nature, bees collect only the most nutritive and healthy pollens. They will pass by poor pollen. As the bees bring the pollen into the hive, some of it will fall off their legs onto the bottom of the enclosure. It is this pollen which is considered to be an amazingly high source of potent vitamins, minerals and amino acids, as well as substances that promote longevity and the healing of many ailments. After the bees collect and deposit pollen in the hive, they treat it by adding a small portion of nectar to it. This shapes the pollen into manageable, tiny granules and encloses them in a form that shields them from outside assault and makes them a pure, all-natural, and highly potent life-giving, life-extending food.

Because pollen was discovered to be a rich and balanced source of essential nutrients, it was fed to hundreds of animals over a two-year period by scientist-researcher Dr. Remy Chauvin of the Institute for Bee Culture in Bures-sur-Yvette, France. Reporting to the French Academy of Medicine in 1956, Dr. Chauvin said there were no side effects in the test animals. Furthermore, the use of bee pollen gave the animals increased vitality and improved "powers of reproduction" because of boosted fertility.

Dr. Chauvin then gave bee pollen to a test group of youngsters, adults and elderly people and reported the following:

"Clinical tests involving the administration of pollen to humans revealed best results with chronic constipation. Interesting observations were registered in cases of flatulence as well as colonic infections. Patients suffering from chronic diarrhea which even resisted antibiotic treatment showed improvement. Pollen also produces singular increases in weight and strength during convalescence, and is thus a first-class stimulant.

"The first attempts at its use for symptoms of old age have proven most encouraging. Its administration to anemic children produced a rapid increase in red blood cells. It must be mentioned in addition that absolutely no ill-effects were suffered by the many persons who took pollen regularly over a considerable length of time."

Dr. Chauvin also suggests that bee pollen has a natural antibiotic function. He says he saw it stop the spread of salmonella—germs or microbes responsible for food poisoning. "Pollen has the capacity for regulating intestinal functions as well as the ability to destroy harmful microbes in the digestive region." Scientists state they have seen its effectiveness in destroying harmful intestinal bacteria, especially *Escherichia coli,* and thereby create a form of antibiotic cleansing in the internal organs.

Cancer researchers gave a diet of bee pollen to test animals bred to develop tumors. The scientists reported that bee pollen in supervised amounts apparently could delay and control the appearance of cancerous tumors. (*Journal of the National Cancer Institute,* October 1948).

Alin Caillas, French agriculturist and laureate of the Academy of Agriculture, studied the question of whether bee pollen could be nature's perfect food. Could you live on it exclusively (under dire circumstances) and survive? *Professor Caillas reported that 35 grams of pollen each day would satisfy all needed nutritional requirements for the average person.* He said that as little as 20 grams daily would constitute "a survival diet." Under these circumstances, bee pollen could become a perfect food.

Scientists at the Bonny Laboratories of Geneva, Switzerland, discovered that there is total nutrition in bee pollen. They say: "Generally speaking (there are variations from one type to another) bee pollen contains 35 percent protein, of which approximately half is in the form of free amino acids; that is, materials essential to life, which can be assimilated immediately by the body.

"Further, 40 percent of the content is made up of various forms of sugar, 5 percent is fats, 3 percent is minerals and oligo-elements (carriers of calcium, phosphorous, magnesium, iron, copper manganese, etc.), 3 to 4 percent moisture (water) totaling about 86 percent. The remainder is composed of trace elements, only a few of which have been identified (amines, nicotinic acid, pantothenic acid, folic acid, biotin, cyanocobalamin).

"We find the B complex vitamins in large quantities and also vitamins A, C, D and E. The pigments which give the pollen its color have been isolated. This coloring, varying between light cream and blue-black depending on origin, covers every shade of the full spectrum. Uncounted diatase (also known as diastase, an enzyme) and hormone components, growth-producers and antibiotics complete this already *extraordinarily* versatile food. In addition, there is no doubt that bee pollen contains other active ingredients not yet known.

*"It is evident that pollen's content of elements important to life is extremely high. In many respects it exceeds the content of yeast, sprouted grain and royal jelly, which are known as being extremely vitalizing."*

Reports from Europe indicate that members of the USSR's ice hockey teams, as well as many of its Olympic medal winners, have been longtime partakers of bee pollen as an energizer.

According to Soviet scientists, pollen is a highly concentrated source of essential elements which seem to be the most complete food in nature. It contains all water-soluble vitamins (especially high in B and C), ten amino acids, twenty-seven minerals (including calcium, magnesium, zinc, copper and iron), trace elements and different enzymes. It is believed that weight for weight, bee pollen contains more protein than accepted sources such as meat, fish, eggs and dairy products.

In Norse mythology, the secret of eternal life of the gods was in the food they ate—ambrosia. This ambrosia was a delicious-tasting combination of honey as well as beebread—another name for the pollen stored up in honeycomb cells. By eating this ambrosia, or bee pollen, the gods could live forever. In the days of ancient Greece and Rome, pollen was considered a staple food for athletes as well as all others who wanted to enjoy greater vigor and a longer lasting, youthful life. In ancient times, all honey was wild honey and it was eaten with the comb. In modern times, the pollen has been gathered separately and is available in health food stores and many pharmacies in the form of tablets as well as powder.

Dr. Naum Petrowitsch Joirisch, member of the Academy of Science in the USSR, a scientist with the department of physiology at the Far East Institute of the Soviet Academy of Science in Vladivostok, researched bee pollen and discovered that it has an amazingly high concentrate of health-boosting powers. Writing in *Bees in the Service of Humanity* (published in 1975 by Nauka in Moscow), Dr. Joirisch tells of these powers of bee pollen:

"Pollen is one of the original treasure houses for our nutrition and our medicine. Each grain of pollen contains protein, fats, carbohydrates, vitamins, ferments (enzymes), minerals, hormones *and every other important substance necessary to a living organism.*

"Pollen protein contains ten different amino acids; some are replaceable, some are not. Pollen is also a natural concentrate of nearly all natural vitamins: each grain contains vitamins A, B-complex, C, D, E as well as rutin.

"Pollen contains very important enzymes for the human organism—they take part as biological catalysts. From some kinds of plants, pollen contains estrogen and androgen (hormones) as well as numerous bio-elements, minerals such as calcium, magnesium, copper, iron, phosphorous, chlorine, sulphur, silicon and many other trace elements.

"For the existence of the bee colony, pollen is of the utmost importance. If there is not enough pollen in the hive, the queen stops reproducing. The worker bees make no more wax or combs—the colony dies."

Dr. Joirisch then says that not only was the regular eating of honey and pollen beneficial to the long-living beekeepers studied in the USSR, "but also the blossom dust content of the air seems to have an effect on the long life of the beekeepers. As a biological stimulant, the effect of pollen deserves special attention in the aging organism. Bulgarian scientists think that pollen improves the physical and emotional well-being of old people. After taking pollen, lifeless and aging skin becomes firm and smooth again. For this reason pollen is already being used as a medical cosmetic.

"Beekeepers inhale pollen just by breathing and this seems to create a feeling of inner peace and balance."

Professor Joirisch then adds: "This existence of the

most important and necessary vitamins in pollen makes it one of the most universal natural remedies. For hundreds of years, pollen has existed in every day medicine as a remedy with many healing properties. It is able to help regulate and control blood pressure; it can bring down high blood pressure.

"Other studies proved that pollen together with honey cured illnesses of the nervous and endocrinological systems. In other tests . . . pollen was able to reduce and eliminate disease bacteria in subjects. This points to the antibiotic success of pollen.

"A healing effect was shown where there was pernicious anemia and disturbances of the intestinal functions such as colitis, chronic constipation.

"Finally, it was discovered that pollen as a supplement increases the appetite and work performance. Of great importance is the immediate benefit of pollen to the blood. Pollen increases the content of hemoglobin (red coloring matter of the bloodstream) and also of erythrocytes (red blood cell occurring in bone marrow) in cases of anemia.

"Particularly interesting were results obtained by the French scientist, Dr. L. Perin, who treated youngsters suffering from anemia. One teaspoonful of pollen each day for breakfast showed that the number of erythrocytes in the blood of the children increased by nearly 300,000 per cubic millimeter."

Professor Joirisch explains that pollen is a marvelous biological stimulant. It stimulates the regeneration in the organism; it slows down aging. The health and emotional well-being of aging people improve with pollen. There are also improvements in the endocrinological (hormonal) system.

### Basics About Beekeeping

Let us take a closer look at the bee colony and see how honey and bee pollen are harvested and made ready for your use.

Honey bees are social insects. This means that they live together in a colony and depend on each other for survival. Most of the bees in a colony are workers (females). Some are drones (males), whose only function is to mate with the queen bee. Usually, there is one queen bee in the colony; she lays the eggs that maintain or increase the colony's population.

Worker bees number up to sixty thousand, depending on the egg-laying ability of the colony queen, the space available in the hive for expansion and the incoming food supply. Worker bees live about six weeks. They collect food and water for the entire colony, do the housework and guard the hive against intruders. They also "air-condition" the hive and maintain a constant hive temperature and humidity—whatever the conditions outside. Although worker bees do not mate, they may lay eggs if the colony loses its queen. But their eggs will not keep up the colony population, because they develop only into drones.

The number of drones in a colony varies with the season of the year. There may be none during the winter, but several hundred during the summer. They are driven out of the hive in the fall, when worker bees can no longer collect food.

The queen bee normally flies from the hive when she

is about a week old and mates in the air with several drones. When she returns to the hive, she begins to lay eggs. During her lifetime she lays thousands of eggs— sometimes as many as a thousand in a day. She puts each egg into a separate cell of the honeycomb.

Three days after an egg is laid, it hatches into a larva. Worker bee "nursemaids" feed and care for the larva, for six days. Then they seal the cell. Inside the honeycomb cell, the larva transforms into a pupa. Twenty-one days from the day the egg was laid, an adult bee chews its way out of the cell.

Bees cannot make honey without nectar, a liquid, sugary substance produced by flowers. It is the raw material of honey and the bees' main source of food. The color and flavor of honey depend on the kinds of plants that bees collect nectar from. Honey may be colorless, amber or even reddish; its flavor can range from mild to strong.

As worker bees gather nectar from flowers, tiny particles of pollen stick to their bodies and are accumulated in pellets on their hind legs. This pollen is carried back to the hive, where the bees store it as beebread in the cells of the honeycomb. Later, worker bees in the hive consume the beebread and its nutrients are converted into larval food by special glands in the heads of the "nursemaids." (The few young larvae selected by the workers to become new queens are fed a greater amount of an enriched larval food commonly called royal jelly.)

Pollen, therefore, is necessary for producing new bees. An average-size colony of bees uses about a hundred pounds of pollen each year. Many wild flowers, ornamentals, weeds, shrubs and trees provide pollen.

*How Bees Make Honey and Wax.* The nectar that bees collect is generally half to three-fourths water. After nectar is carried into the hive, the bees evaporate most of the water from it. While the water is being evaporated, enzymes change the nectar into honey. Then the bees seal the honey into cells of the honeycomb.

Beeswax begins as a liquid made by glands on the underside of the worker bee's abdomen. As it is produced, it hardens into tiny wax scales. Worker bees then use this wax to build the honeycomb.

Beekeepers often provide their bees with honeycomb foundation made of sheets of beeswax. This foundation fits into hive frames and becomes the base of the honeycomb. It enables bees to speed up comb construction, and it provides a pattern for building a straight and easy-to-remove honeycomb.

The tiny bee is a source of power. A bee will carry as much as its own weight in pollen, taking it back every day to the hive to feed the bee larvae and all-important queen. Pollen consists of millions of tiny grains with very delicate forms and designs representing the specific flower from which it comes. Pollination is the transfer of pollen from the anther of a flower to the stigma of a pistil of another flower; there it reaches the ovary, where fertilization occurs. From here, the reproductive seeds are developed. Without this transfer of pollen, without the pollen itself, plant life and most growth could perish.

# CHAPTER 3

## *THE CANCER-FIGHTING*
## *ELEMENTS IN BEE POLLEN*

As a thief of life, cancer is seizing more and more victims with the passing of the years. Even though there have been many medical advances in treating this disease, a single cure has eluded the researchers. Cancer is a disorder of cell growth. It begins in a group of cells (or a single cell) that divide regardless of need. Cancer is a parasite formed within the person's own tissues. It is a family or tribe of cells that has become alienated from its neighbors; it no longer serves as a part of the harmonious community of cells that makes a healthy body.

Cancer is not subject to the normal control of nerves and hormones. It draws on the available supply of nourishment but gives nothing in return. Because cancer is not subject to any control, because cancer cells have nothing to do but reproduce themselves, in time they will outnumber the healthy cells. Unchecked, they will spread beyond the limits of their original organ, being carried in lymph vessels or veins to other parts of the body where they may form metastases (sites where cancer is lodged and then spreads to other locations throughout the body).

In brief, cancer is an alteration in the behavior of cells in response to various harmful factors. Some of these factors are known, many others are unknown.

Often cancer is undetected until there is a routine examination. This emphasizes the need for yearly checkups by the physician who can discover possible threats of cancer. Often, some outward symptoms are considered warning signals that should be brought to the doctor's attention without delay. Such warning signals, listed by the American Cancer Society, are these:

1. Any sore that does not heal
2. A lump or thickening in the breast or elsewhere
3. Unusual bleeding or discharge
4. Any change in a wart or mole
5. Persistent indigestion or difficulty in swallowing
6. Persistent hoarseness or cough
7. Any change in normal bowel habits

Because cancer is on the increase and claiming more and more lives, researchers are seeking any available program or remedy that will offer prevention or healing in one degree or another. It is possible that bee pollen can control this runaway cellular growth. In one such report, appearing in the *Journal of the National Cancer Institute* (October 1948, pp. 119-23), a group of test mice were subjected to the growth of cancerous tumors, then fed bee pollen. Cellular proliferation halted.

In this report, prepared by William Robinson, U.S. Department of Agriculture researcher with its Bureau of Entomology, the following facts are cited:

"In some preliminary experiments, it was observed that the addition of pollen to the food of mice of the $C_3H$ strain (a form of cancer) delayed the appearance of spontaneous mammary (breast) tumors eight to ten weeks."

The mice were then given bee pollen in various amounts, and records were kept. Says this official report, "The pollen was supplied by the Division of Bee Culture, of the Bureau of Entomology and Plant Quarantine of the U.S. Department of Agriculture, and was the *bee-gathered type*. Bees gather pollen from many species of plants as an essential food for their young. They carry it into the hives in pellet form, about 100 to the gram, and each pellet contains about 500,000 pollen.

"The pellets are recovered by means of a trap which causes the bees to drop the pellets into a container. In this way, about 30 pounds of pellets can be obtained annually per hive. The pollen used was collected in Wisconsin and California. It was mixed and stored at a temperature of about 4° C. or 36° F.

"The pollen was prepared for use by grinding 1 gram of pellets in a mortar with 50 milliliters of distilled water, a small amount of the water being used at first to form a thin paste, and the remainder was then added. For the sake of uniformity, this stock suspen-

sion was used within one-half hour of grinding to avoid
the possibility that extraction would take place.

"The food was pollinized as follows: 6 pounds of
powdered food (Purina Laboratory Chow ground to
powder form in a food grinder) was placed in a large
food mixer. The required amount of pollen suspension
was drawn up into a graduated pipette. Because the
suspension settles rapidly, it had to be stirred while
being drawn up.

"The foods were then placed in plainly marked containers, ready for use" by the test animals.

For a series of many weeks, the cancerous mice were
fed this pollen food. Tests were made regularly. "In the
preliminary tests, *an apparent delay in the development
of mammary tumors occurred in the mice ingesting
small amounts of pollen* (the male gamete of plants
being used because of availability)."

A control group of test mice was set up and it was
found that without being given the pollen food, their
tumors increased and did not halt.

"These results indicate that under suitable conditions, the development of mammary tumors in the $C_3H$
mice can be influenced by ingestion of pollinized food.
It is suggested that the use of extracted and standard-
ized active principle from pollen might produce greater
postponement.

*"These experiments were based upon the postulation
that pollen contains an anti-carcinogenic principle that
can be added to the food."*

The use of pollen must be regulated according to
strength as well as to frequency and duration of feeding. The researcher says, "This finding indicates that

the dosage of pollen could be made too strong or that the pollen feeding might be started too early, and could thus nullify the postponement effect." Therefore, in the test mice, various dosages were given to different groups to determine effective rates. "Early indications suggest that a weaker pollen diet was more likely to result in postponement of tumors." This suggests that bee pollen is very powerful and so potent that even a weak or *small amount* is vigorous enough to affect the growth of cancerous tumors.

Bee pollen is often chosen as a healer over honey because there is a difference. Carried back to the hive, pollen becomes combined with honey. These honey scraps or dark residues gather at the bottom of the hive. Therefore, *pure honey is devoid of these important honey scraps or pollen.* While pure honey is a potent vitamin-mineral food, it is pollen that is preferred by researchers as a means of health building and cancer fighting because it contains a high concentration of valuable nutrients and substances not found in honey. Pollen appears to be a miracle food in the battle against cancer.

# CHAPTER 4

## HOW BEE POLLEN CAN HELP YOU LIVE LONGER

In *Bees in the Service of Humanity,*
Dr. Joirisch says that bee pollen "contains highly
prophylactic and therapeutic properties. It is a strong
biological stimulant (with) regenerative powers for the
organism." He found that older people who took regular
amounts of raw bee pollen "seemed to enjoy better res-
toration of morale, a sense of emotional well-being and
actual physical health." The skin that was formerly aging now started to become rejuvenated. Dr. Joirisch
believes that bee pollen could help extend the life span
and also create an appearance of better and healthier
youth.

Bee pollen is high in aspartic acid, an amino acid
that is able to stimulate the glands to promote a feeling
of bodily rejuvenation. It also contains still other potent rejuvenating factors such as sterines, steroid hor-

mone substances as well as gonadotropic hormones—
plant hormones similar to the gonadotropin secreted by
the pituitary to stimulate the reproductive glands. These
substances alert a sluggish metabolic process so that internal rejuvenation is possible through glandular awak-
ening. This will help add years to the life span.

The long-living peoples of Abkhasia frequently enjoy a life span that goes over a hundred. Abkhasia is
one of the Soviet Republics in the Russian Caucasus
region. The people of Abkhasia do more than just eat
honey, which is considered a daily food. They are a
thrifty people, and knowing that no one would buy the
debris, the honey scrap or the pollen found in the bottom of the beehive, they eat it rather than let it go to
waste. Factors in this pollen appear to give the
Abkhasian people an enviably long life span, yet they
are not aware of its longevity value.

Pollen is a highly potent, concentrated form of protein—at least 35 percent protein. About half of this
amount is in the form of free amino acids which are
immediately used by the body for rebuilding and rejuvenation. Some people have a metabolism so sluggish
that the protein isn't transformed into usable amino
acids, and body health declines. But when pollen is
eaten, the free amino acids require almost no metabolism and are speedily assimilated, no matter how weak
the digestive system.

Researcher Dr. Sula Benet went to Abkhasia and reported (*The New York Times*, December 25, 1972)
hearing one ninety-nine-year-old man tell his doctor,
"It isn't time to die yet. I am needed by my children
and grandchildren. It isn't bad in this world—except

that I can't turn the earth over and it has become difficult to climb trees." At age ninety-nine, he was vigorous, alert and healthy.

Researchers found that the pollen-eating Abkhasians enjoy sex well up into their so-called later years, and that many men had vigorous sexual potency long after the age of 70. One 102-year-old Abkhasian said he had "a desire for my wife but no strength." Another man had nine children; the last one was born when he was 100 years of age. Reportedly 119, he is said to have a healthy libido and potency. As for women, many can bear children even in their late fifties. It is estimated that the women don't enter the menopause till after the age of 55.

Two of the greatest gerontologists of the USSR, Professors Nikita Mankovsky and D. G. Chebotarev, have also found that pollen is able to cause self-renewal or rejuvenation and add years to the life span. They feel that rejuvenation of body cells can be stimulated by the administration of polyvitamins, micro-elements, enzymes and amino acids to form new tissues. These substances are found in bee pollen, which is praised by the USSR scientists as having the ability to create a form of internal-external rejuvenation as well as life extension.

If you introduce hormones into your system, you have an opportunity for adding many years of good health to your life. Pollen contains such cell-feeding hormones. According to E. Kvanta, a Swedish researcher, as reported in *Acta Chemica Scandinavia* (V 22, no. 7 [1968]: 216–65), "The presence of sterols or hormones in pollen from various plants has been described." According to various reports, the hormones in pollen would appear to stimulate the body's sluggish glands and to act as a supplement to make up for any endocrine deficiency. This helps wake up the so-called weak glands and supercharge the body with youthful vitality and a longer life span.

Pollen contains twenty-two basic elements. The human body is composed of twenty-two elements which are found in only one food—bee pollen. When pollen enters your digestive system, its twenty-two elements immediately start to regulate and invigorate metabolism by supplying any missing substances, such as enzymes not provided by other foods. Pollen elements then help control the destructive reaction of toxins, pollutants and drugs. They shield the body from the assault that may cause premature aging and loss of precious years of life. As such, the pollen elements rejuvenate body cells and add more vigorous years to your allotted time.

Ingredients in bee pollen activate body processes to prevent aging caused by sluggishness. Some of these life-extending ingredients are:

*Vitamins.* All known vitamins are present in a highly concentrated package to promote the various processes of the body, so that cell-tissue growth continues at a healthy rate.

*Glucosides.* These are natural sugars that combine with both the natural amount of fructose and glucose to create body energy and vitality.

*Enzymes.* Pollen contains many enzymes such as phosphatase, amylase and diastase which are needed to promote better metabolism and fermentation and transform food into youth-building elements. Enzymes will also use amino acids in the pollen and in the body for the rebuilding of body organs and revitalization of processes.

*Hormones.* Pollen contains sterols or plant hormones which can often take up the slack caused by diminishing endocrine activity. They also tend to activate the body glands and help them release a healthy supply of natural hormones for youthful longevity.

*Antibiotic Factors.* These substances found in bee pollen create a regulatory action on the intestinal region, produce improved blood health, calm and soothe the body through a healthy neuromuscular reaction. Toxic wastes and poisons are then neutralized through the antibiotic or disinfecting reaction of the pollen.

*Rutin.* This is a glucoside in bee pollen that increases the resistance of the capillary walls to infectious poisons. Pollen rutin will also help stabilize metabolism, which will improve respiration, emotional health and heart rhythm. It cuts down the time of bleeding so there is better healing and coagulation of the blood, and will reinforce the contraction of the heart and regulate its rhythm, which is most beneficial for heart health. Pollen rutin helps control hypertension by regulating the blood flow and soothing the nervous system.

Other life-giving benefits of bee pollen are:

1. Gives to your body those missing elements that will create total health
2. Reestablishes the healthy action of bodily functions

which could otherwise be deficient and cause premature aging
3. Stimulates and increases vital energy, needed for a longer life span
4. Acts as a tonic, stimulates the body, cleanses the organism so that it can respond with more youth-building benefits

As mentioned earlier, Dr. Naum Joirisch feels that pollen as well as pollen dust that is inhaled could prolong life. In his *Bees in the Service of Humanity*, Dr. Joirisch says:

". . . the centenarian beekeepers are always surrounded by pollen-contained air near their bees. They inhale the tiny pollen grains; the pollen develops its long-life 'youth-giving' effect in the bodies of the beekeepers. We also examined a gerontologist-colleague, Professor Dr. Grigorij Pizchelauri. This scientist has, for many years, been researching the reasons why so many mountain inhabitants in the Caucasus reach one hundred and more. He discovered that a high number of the centenarians lived around the Black Sea and Caspian Sea in bee-populated areas. They took honey and pollen daily. They also breathed in the pollen 'dust' and this is believed to give them added years. Prof. Dr. Pizchelauri is also healthy and alert because he takes both honey and pollen daily."

# CHAPTER 5

## THE POLLEN POWER BEHIND ATHLETES

In ancient days, bee pollen was the "ambrosia of the gods" and was a staple for Greek athletes girding their loins for Olympics. This same ambrosia is now being fed to Olympian athletes who then go on to become winners, as in days of yore.

The Olympic athletes have discovered that they can improve their performances by taking bee pollen tablets. In particular, Finland trained over a thousand young men and women for the 1976 Olympics by giving them good food along with pollen supplements. These supplements were considered part of their training. The Finnish track coach, Antti Lananaki, told the press in the summer of 1976, "Most of our athletes take the bee pollen food supplement. Our studies show that it significantly improves their performance. There have been no negative results since we began supplying bee pollen to our athletes." Many Finnish runners came away with awards, and it is believed that part of their superior athletic power could be traced to the energizing effect of bee pollen.

Another strong advocate of the use of bee pollen is Lasse Viren, the Finnish star who won the 5000 and 10,000 meter races in 1972 and again in 1976. He, too, attributes his superior athletic vigor to the daily intake of bee pollen.

He takes six to ten tablets a day during training, from four to six tablets during competition.

Steve Riddick, Gold Medalist on the U.S. Relay Team at Montreal in 1976, calls bee pollen "fantastic" and credits it for increasing his recovery power after a hard sprint by 75 percent. "It gives me a lot more energy, too. I used to take honey but this bee pollen is far better. I take three pills a day." He also set an unofficial world's record for the 100 meter dash at a meet in Switzerland in 1975.

As reported in the Long Island, New York newspaper *Newsday,* entertainer Dick Gregory credits his stamina and athletic ability to health foods such as wheat germ and vitamins but especially to bee pollen. "It gives you lightning fast energy that will scare you to death." He says he was able to run fifty miles a day and has this athletic ability because of eating bee pollen along with other health foods. He takes chia seeds because they are one of nature's most nutritious foods. They release energy already locked up in the body. He also takes pumpkin seed oil, garlic capsules, Korean ginseng and even sarsaparilla root, which he finds gives him strength. He also takes kelp. "You could live on kelp. Ninety-eight percent of the things you need are in kelp." But it is bee pollen that gives him the athletic stamina he needs.

Many coaches as well as athletes use bee pollen, which they regard as energy in a capsule. As reported in *Let's Live* (July 1976), here are some of the athletic-boosting benefits of this natural food:

After his track team had been given bee pollen for four months, trainer Jack Gimmler at St. John's University, Queens, New York, was so convinced of the performance of his athletes that he was able to persuade the university to underwrite a year's supply for sixty athletes—including track, basketball and swimming.

At Seton Hall University in New Jersey, athletes were put on a three-month program of taking bee pollen. Coach John Moon was able to build up their vigor so that the athletes set a U.S. indoor track record for the mile relay in Detroit. Later, the same bee-pollen-energized athletes took top honors at the Metropolitan Intercollegiate Indoor Track and Field Championships at Princeton.

Trainer Doug Boyd at Fairleigh Dickinson University in Rutherford, New Jersey, gives bee pollen to his athletes who have many winning scores to their credit.

Coach Tommy Smith at Oberlin in Ohio also gives bee pollen to his budding athletes. More research is being conducted to determine whether this energizing food should be given to athletes throughout the country, and the world.

"Athletes as diverse as Olympic distance runners and professional basketball players are popping tablets of pollen at the rate of five or 10 a day," says *The New York Times* (February 6, 1977). "John Williamson, the high-scoring guard traded by the Nets to Indiana this week, says his 10 tablets a day give him this burst of energy on the court he did not even know he had."

Dr. Roger Morse, professor of apiculture at Cornell University, says, "People have been eating bee pollen for hundreds of years. It's a good, rich source of protein."

Dr. Charles W. Turner, head trainer for Long Island University, traveled throughout the world and came upon bee pollen in 1973 while in Europe. (Dr. Turner reached the young age of eighty-two in 1977.) He feels bee pollen does provide energy and vigor for athletes. He also uses bee pollen as a poultice to reduce swelling of the limbs that frequently occurs among athletes. He dissolves pollen pellets in warm tap water until they form an infusion. He dips a towel in the mixture and applies it to the injured region. Dr. Turner says, "I've seen swelling go down a half inch in twenty minutes because of this pollen poultice. I've seen results on all but two of the 189 knees, ankles and the like that were given this pollen poultice."

A Long Island University gymnast, Brigitte Bouchereau, underwent cartilage surgery on her knees. She went on a bee pollen program, both internal and external (in the form of a poultice), and says, "I've improved a lot. My knees are like 100 percent better."

Dr. Turner says, "I know I'll have trouble with the medical people on this. There are too many big shots among doctors. They don't have time to listen to small cases. If the treatment worked only 50 percent of the time, they'd accept it.

"We are pollen people. We believe in it. . . . We want to get a certain amount of medical men involved in the experiments, but we don't feel we're quite ready yet."

At age thirty-seven, George Stillman was able to run fifty-two and a half miles from the New York side of the George Washington Bridge to Middletown Township, New Jersey, for a time span of seven hours and forty minutes, in January 1977. This former Asbury Park (New Jersey) High School and University of Maryland athlete was able to run with good mental and physical stamina, during severe weather, *subsisting exclusively on just one food item—bee pollen*. Two aides followed him via automobile and kept him energized with bee pollen pellets.

As reported in the *Asbury Park Press* (January 23, 1977), George Stillman originally planned this special run on December 26, 1976, as his parting salute to the Bicentennial year and American awareness of physical fitness.

But there was a very heavy snow and ice storm, so he had to postpone this 52½-mile run until January 16, 1977. Even so, when this bee-pollen-nourished athlete went across the George Washington Bridge, he was greeted by light snow flurries in twenty-four-degree weather . . . hardly a climate conducive to running, especially for a man of thirty-seven, and considered to be out of his prime by current youthful standards. But George Stillman would not be delayed. He started to run, even though there were frozen roadways and slippery conditions. He started to slow in a semijog, then went to an occasional speed walk.

"The temperature was still dropping as I got past the Amboys. My muscles started to pull in the thighs and the back. And I have a lower left lumbar condition to start off with." Soon, he said, he had "cold and stiffness through my arms, legs and shoulders. The whole left side of me seemed strained." But he persisted. Stillman credits his energy and vitality in being able to complete the 52½-mile run in bad weather because of his mental alertness and also the bee pollen.

Les Wallach, a coach at Rutgers University, gave bee pollen to his track athletes over a period of time. The runners went on to win the New Jersey cross-country championship for the first time. In November 1976, the cross-country team won the Metropolitan Intercollegiate Cross-Country Championship in New York. After forty-eight years of running *without winning a single title*, the athletes started to gather up championships. Coach Wallach, as reported in the *New Brunswick* (N.J.) *Home News* (November 8, 1976), attributed their sudden winning streak to good training as well as to bee pollen. Said Coach Wallach:

"No one makes any claims that bee pollen is beneficial, but I think that it is. I take it myself. I feel great. I've had no head colds, a lot more vitality and I find I am sleeping more restfully.

"Others have told me of claims for bee pollen. I heard about it after the 1972 Olympics, recommended them for my track team to add nutrients because I felt they might not be eating the proper foods while carrying a heavy workload as students and athletes."

## Pollen Power Behind Athletes

Bee pollen is especially rich in a potent member of the B-complex vitamin group, namely, pantothenic acid, which has a key role in metabolism, for antibody formation and also for the stimulus of the nervous system. This vitamin helps the body build resistance to stress and has a healthy and natural influence on the production of the adrenal-cortical hormones. When the glandular system is adequately nourished with sufficient pantothenic acid as found in bee pollen, it does create a powerhouse of vitality and energy. This may be one of the many reasons why it is able to stimulate athletes of different ages to transform them from average runners to champions.

### Athletic Coach Cheers Bee Pollen

Tom McNab, who has been the official national athletics coach to the British athletic teams, is responsible for the training of members of the national team and for ensuring that they consume a diet suitable for their athletic activities.

Coach McNab says, "I frequently test food supplements alleged by their manufacturers to assist athletes in reaching their optimum physical condition. To test the efficacy of one of these supplements, I ask a number of athletes training under either my supervision or that of other coaches to take the supplement in accordance with the manufacturer's recommendations. I then carefully monitor the athletic performance of the athletes to see whether any improvement in their ability results from taking the product tested.

"In October, 1973, I was asked to test the efficacy of a bee pollen product. I was initially skeptical of the results likely to be obtained by use of this product. However, I asked five athletes training under me to take bee pollen in accordance with the manufacturer's directions; that is, one to three pills a day. Within a period of 12 months, the athletic performance of all of the five athletes taking bee pollen had substantially improved."

Here are the results:

The best performance of a female hurdler, age twenty-eight, prior to taking bee pollen was 13.3 seconds. After taking the pollen, training levels rose immediately. She improved to 12.9 seconds and won a Commonwealth Games Gold Medal.

When a male decathlete, age eighteen, started taking bee pollen, his body weight went up eight pounds, and within four weeks, there was a big rise in his weight-training capacity. Personal performances improved in training.

Before taking bee pollen, the best performance of a twenty-five-year-old female hurdler was 14.1 seconds. Soon she improved to 13.6 seconds and achieved a good position in the British team. There was a noticeable improvement in her work rate.

Before taking bee pollen, the best performance of a male javelin thrower, age twenty-three, was 210 feet. After taking bee pollen, he improved to 235 feet 6 inches. Again, a big improvement in work rate, weight and muscle mass was noted.

Before taking bee pollen, the best performance of a twenty-four-year-old male hurdler was 51.8 seconds. After taking bee pollen, he improved to 50.7 seconds. He gained a well-deserved place in the Commonwealth

Games Team. He considers bee pollen to be an essential part of his training diet.

Coach Tom McNab concludes: "The main value of bee pollen is not just in its direct effect upon performance, but rather in its apparent effect upon training levels. This rise in training levels enables more work to be done, more skill to be acquired and more muscle to be developed.

"The effect of bee pollen is particularly notable in underweight athletes. Both the javelin thrower and the decathlete noted an immediate (that is, within two weeks) rise in bodyweight and lean muscle mass.

"It is usually presumptuous to ascribe improvement to any single factor. However, I believe that bee pollen has had a significant effect on the cases described, especially on the last-named male hurdler, whose work rate improvement was dramatic.

"A beneficial side effect, which I attribute to bee pollen has been the diminution of the number of colds which the athletes have experienced. Freedom from such complaints is a major factor in any training program.

"I conclude that bee pollen is the most effective revitalizing food supplement available to athletes today of all the food supplements which I have tested."

Mr. McNab said that, among the track and field athletes he trained for the Olympics, "At least 90 percent of our athletes are taking bee pollen tablets daily. Most claim that it improves their performance, and gives them greater stamina and more energy."

To boost your own stamina and energy, to help revitalize your body and mind so that you can enjoy the best that life has to offer you, take bee pollen daily. You may not become a Gold Medal champion or Olympic winner, but you will feel like one. Life will then become well worth living.

# CHAPTER 6

## HOW BEE POLLEN IMPROVES DIGESTION

Bee pollen is a natural way to help correct problems of the digestive system and restore a feeling of youthfulness to this entire region. Because pollen consists of an inverted sugar, it does not ferment or "sour" in the digestive tract. It is speedily absorbed, helps keep out bacterial invasion and has a demulcent (soothing) effect on irritated or inflamed intestines. By its natural lubricating power and natural fatty acid content, bee pollen stimulates sluggish peristalsis, resulting in regularity without the need for laxatives and in elimination of bulk with less strain.

Bee pollen is a rapidly acting source of muscular energy and promotes a restorative reaction to the digestive system. The pollen will activate digestive muscles so that they are able to consume four times as much

energy-creating glycogen as when at rest, thus invigorating the digestive system.

When bee pollen is taken by itself, without food, it
appears to work unhindered in correcting errors of metabolism which may be involved in unhealthy weight
gain. Here is how this works to control weight:

Sugars and fats are both energy-providing and car-
bon-containing foods; when they combine with oxygen,
they burn up to produce energy. Sugars are higher in
carbon elements; they are flammable and produce this
energy very quickly. Fats are lower in carbon and oxygen elements than sugars. Therefore, fats are metabo-
lized slower because their function is to supply reserve
energy. Fats need more oxygen to be set afire to be put
into reserve for future use.

When bee pollen inverted sugars are taken into your
digestive system, there is a speedy combustion. The
fats will burn with the help of oxygen produced by
their "fire." This causes a speedy increase in the rate of
sugar metabolism and there is an increased rate of
calorie burning and consequent weight loss. It is bee
pollen which causes this internal reaction. It is the
natural way to improve metabolism and help control
and take off weight.

Those who have put much store in the effects of lactic acid would do well to consider bee pollen as a com-
plementary source of digestive healing. So says Dr.
Paavo O. Airola in *Health Secrets From Europe*:

"It has been suggested that Bulgarians, Rumanians,
Russians and other East European peoples known for
their enviable record of longevity have to thank *lactic
acid* for their excellent health and youthful vitality.

Their diets are high in soured foods (rich in lactic acid) such as sour milk, yogurt, black sourdough bread, sauerkraut and the like. Lactic acid has a beneficial anti-putrefactive effect on the intestines and keeps the digestive tract in good health.

"Probably the most beneficial effect of pollen is that, taken internally, *it quickly produces the same anti-putrefactive effect as lactic acid foods, and thus contributes to a healthy digestive system and good assimilation of nutrients—absolute prerequisites for good health and long life.*"

A dramatic case of the digestive-satisfying powers of bee pollen is offered by U.S. Air Force Lieutenant Colonel Thomas J. Tretheway. As reported in *The Golden Pollen* (Yakima, Wash.: Yakima Binding and Printing Company, 1960), during World War II, this paratrooper escaped from a Japanese prison camp in Burma. Natives helped Tretheway escape. They were interested in traveling speedily so did not weigh themselves down with food. Instead, whenever they came to a stream, they would skim floating pollen off the water, offer a good portion to Tretheway and eat much of it themselves. Tretheway says they went through the rigors of jungle traveling and ate absolutely nothing but pollen. This satisfied them. All were healthy, energetic and youthful. He even regained weight he lost in prison camp on a sole diet of bee pollen.

Colonel Tretheway reported that he and the natives either ate the pollen by itself or else they would mix it with honey and eat it in the form of a cake. He says, "All of them were tall, slender, had perfect teeth. Youngsters and adults appeared to be in perfect health on a staple diet of pollen. I, too, felt healthy from this exclusive and sole fare."

Tretheway said that when he developed gangrene-like feet, the natives would coat his wounds with a poultice of pollen and honey, which promoted speedy healing. When Tretheway eventually made it to safety in Calcutta, he was told by a British physician that he had to thank pollen and honey because they saved his feet . . . and his life!

Later, Tretheway told his superiors that pollen was such a complete or all-purpose or "perfect" food that it was an excellent survival food—someone could live on it and remain in good digestive health and survive even in the total absence of all other food.

# CHAPTER 7

## HEAL YOUR ALLERGIES WITH BEE POLLEN

Many allergies, such as asthma or hay fever, are caused by pollen introduced into the respiratory system. But scientists have found that bee pollen can help build immunity and that there is a difference between inhaled pollen and the bee pollen product.

Allergies are caused generally by breathing in the anemophilous pollens which are carried by the wind. To help build a form of natural immunity, your body requires a supply of entomophilous pollens (gathered by the bees from a variety of different blossoms) that will act as a barrier or shield against the windborne and inhaled pollens that are responsible for your allergic reaction. The bee-collected pollens are often very sticky and heavy and cannot be carried by the wind. These pollens are healing because when the bees form them into pellets, they add a little nectar and saliva. This neutralizes and déstroys any allergic principle (if one existed) and makes bee pollen a respiratory-strengthening food that can help heal and even prevent allergies. By taking one teaspoon of bee pollen daily, resistance to wind-carried pollen is slowly built up and the sensitivity to allergy is reduced. Gradually, your body builds up a shield to insulate you from the irritating effects of wind-carried pollen.

The ability of bee pollen to immunize the body against allergies was reported in the *Florida Farmers Bulletin* (October 15, 1969) under the title, "Doctors Recommend Raw Honey Treatment for Allergies":

"An Oklahoma allergist told a meeting of 150 beekeepers that raw honey is an effective treatment for 90 percent of all allergies. Dr. William G. Peterson, an allergist from Ada, Oklahoma, said he now has 22,000 patients across the nation who are using raw honey—along with more customary medication—to relieve allergic symptoms.

" 'It must be raw honey, because raw honey contains all the pollen, dust, and molds that cause 90 percent of all allergies. What happens is that the patient builds up an immunity to the pollen, dust or mold that is causing his trouble in the first place,' " Dr. Peterson told the meeting of the Oklahoma Beekeepers Association.

" 'The raw honey must not be strained, not even through a cloth. I know the customer wants good, clear, strained, filtered honey and that's fine, but for health reasons, raw honey is what we need.

" 'Along with myself, there are 20 doctors at my clinic in Ada who normally prescribe a daily teaspoon of raw honey. This honey treatment continues even after the allergy is under control.' "

This form of natural immunity is made possible by the traces of pollens, dust and molds found in raw honey. However, pure bee pollen is more concentrated and contains a very potent power in causing self-immunity against allergies. Therefore, while raw honey is excellent, pollen should also be taken regularly as a highly concentrated source of self-immunization.

If you have an allergy, you are tested by your doctor to discover the cause. Once the doctor finds out the reason you are sensitive or determines the substance responsible for giving you such symptoms as chills, itching, fever, sniffles, etc., then he will inject that particular offender in minute amounts into your bloodstream. This builds up resistance to the offender. Sometimes, this calls for lifetime injections, since your body will constantly use up and remove the injected serum and it must be replaced. Often, too, there are side effects felt from these injections.

Writing in *Bee Pollen, Miracle Food*, Felix Murat says:

"In France—and this is a practice that originated in the United States—doctors inject an extract from pollen to immunize the allergic person.

"A doctor at the Broussais Hospital published the results obtained by this method, which so far was the best treatment known against allergies and especially against its gravest form of bronchial asthma where antihistamine and the other usual treatments did not help.

"The treatment consists of repeated injections from

February 15 to July 15, starting with two injections weekly and ending with one.

"The only inconvenience of this method is that at times and on certain individuals it provokes violent reactions. It is absolutely indispensable that the injections are administered by a doctor, and the doctor must closely supervise the state of his patient for at least one hour after the injection.

"The trouble, however, is that most ill persons are impatient, they think that the trouble will disappear overnight. They forget that these innumerable problems (allergies) took a long time to develop to the point of becoming noticeable; it will take time to bring them under control."

D. S. Jarvis, M.D., writing in *Folk Medicine*, says, "If honeycomb cappings (which are prime sources of pollen) are chewed once each day for one month before the expected hay fever date, the hay fever will not appear or will be mild in character."

Writing in the *American Bee Journal* (December 1950), Dr. Jarvis extols the benefits of propolis or bee glue (a constituent of comb honey) which he says "has a special action on the breathing tract . . . it opens the nose, produces a drying effect . . . lessens catarrhal discharge and . . . cough. It is for this . . . effect and the sedative effect on the body as a whole that comb honey with its propolis is used."

For more concentrated pollen there is, as mentioned earlier, pure bee pollen available in tablet or powder form at almost all health stores and many pharmacies, too, which can be taken throughout the year, on a daily basis, and help the body build its own immunity to allergic distress.

Pollen builds immunity this way: Theoretically, a certain portion of the eaten bee pollen does not go through the process of digestion. This portion remains unchanged as it is speedily assimilated into your bloodstream. Since the membrane enclosing each pollen grain is tough, it protects the grain, sustains it and keeps it alive for weeks or even months. Eating bee pollen daily will build up this supply of membrane-protected pollen in the bloodstream. When you breathe in windborne pollen, the reaction will be much milder as your own immunity is strengthened.

Eating bee pollen is similar to being injected with chemicalized pollen by a doctor. The difference is that you nourish your body with *natural* bee pollen, create *natural* immunity, whereas with chemicals, there are risks of side effects and there is also a need for year-after-year regular immunization programs. With daily intake of natural bee pollen, there isn't the inconvenience of injections and your body is not subjected to double trouble of chemicals and windborne pollen. Natural bee pollen will help strengthen the nasal and respiratory passages and boost resistance to offensive pollen.

Writing in *Honey and Your Health*, Bodog F. Beck, M.D., says that his attention "has been repeatedly called to the beneficial effect of honey on hay fever victims. There are many reports that the consumption of honey collected by bees from goldenrod and fireweed will cure hay fever superinduced by the self-same pollen.

"Now comes Dr. George D. McGrew of the Army

Medical Corps of the William Beaumont General Hospital in El Paso, Texas, with a statement that during the hay fever season, thirty-three hay fever sufferers obtained partial or complete relief through the consumption of honey, produced in their vicinity.

"The brood cells contain a considerable amount of bee bread (pollen) stored by the bees for their young and when this is orally administered *it will produce a gradual immunity against the allergic symptoms caused by the same pollen.*

"Dr. McGrew found particular relief for patients when they chewed the honey with the wax of the brood cells. The hospital staff made an alcoholic extract from pollen and administered it in from one- to ten-drop doses, according to the requirements of the patients."

Pollen is a prime source of a form of protein which causes elevation of the gamma globulins of the body. These substances help the body build natural-immunity defense reactions and these offer a shield against allergic distress.

# CHAPTER 8

## CORRECT PROSTATE DISOR-
## DERS WITH BEE POLLEN

The human male is considered to be as young as his prostate gland. It appears to be a link between man and youth. The prostate is closely connected to fertility in the male, and while difficulty with the organ or removal does not necessarily mean sexual impairment or sexual loss, the ability to reproduce is ended and there is a strong psychological effect that may cause the man to feel he is old and that the prime of life has slipped away.

The quest for youth is identical with the quest of potency throughout the history of man. The ancients sought a special food that would give them the secret of eternal youth which is symbolic of eternal potency, fertility and, of course, virility. Legend refers to ambrosia which has already been identified as beebread or pollen. In modern times, pollen has been considered a "youth food" because it reportedly does provide a feeling of energy, vitality and renewed strength, and it has been prescribed as a means of boosting the health of the prostate gland, thereby creating potency and the feeling of "eternal youth."

Let us first take a closer look at the prostate gland and its effect on potency.

*Location.* The prostate gland, one of the male sex organs, is a rounded mass of muscle fibers and smaller glands located immediately below the urinary bladder, surrounding the outlet of the bladder (urethra). It is the size of a walnut and heart-shaped. It encircles the neck of the urethra as it emerges from the bladder.

*Function.* The prostate secretes an alkaline fluid that makes up part of the semen. During ejaculation, both prostatic fluid and seminal fluid are released through the urethra. These fertile fluids cause conception in the female.

*Fertility.* Man is fertile because of the fluid secreted from the prostate gland. A little above and behind the prostate, on either side of the urethra, are situated seminal vesicles or two tiny sacs. These sacs store sperm cells which are produced in the testicles. The sperm cells need to make their way up from the testicles to get into the seminal vesicles, which is nature's assurance that sperm stored therein will be alive, active and make man fertile during sexual intercourse.

*Virility.* The secretions of the prostate gland keep the sperm alive and active so they can fertilize the female ovum (egg), thus making the woman pregnant. Actually, the seminal vesicles do not empty directly into the urethra, but into the prostate. During ejaculation, there is a tightening or contraction of the muscle tissue surrounding these glands. This contraction forces sperm cells into the prostate gland. Here, the cells blend or mix together with the prostatic fluid. This blend is now propelled into the urethra by a series of contractions and then ejaculated through the penis.

*Prostate Disorders.* Although they may happen at any age, problems or disorders of the prostate occur more frequently during the middle years of a man's life. An enlargement of the gland is the basic disorder. Because of this swelling, there is a sensation of pressure at the outlet of the bladder. There is a desire to pass water very frequently; the encroachment on the urethra tends to obstruct the flow of urine and there is difficulty in voiding. At times, it may be difficult or even impossible to empty the bladder totally. This means that some urine remains in the bladder; it becomes infected with bacteria and can injure the bladder and kidneys. Generally, doctors try to bring down the swelling of the prostate but removal of the gland is usually recommended.

In severe situations, there may be cancer of the prostate, which also causes enlargement and infection as well as inflammation.

Any man who has the urge to void frequently should have his prostate examined, as it may be nature's warning signal that something is not right with this organ of fertility-virility.

Herbert R. Kenyon, M.D., writing in *The Prostate Gland*, says that prostatic difficulties should not be ignored or taken lightly in the hopes that they will just go away. Remedial action is important. An enlarged prostate that obstructs the flow of urine can be more than just painful: if neglected, it can be fatal. So Dr. Kenyon urges medical treatment if one or more of these symptoms are noted:

1. Low back pain
2. Blood in the seminal fluid or urine
3. An abnormal or unhealthy acceleration of sexual desire or frequently recurring erections that come without any special stimulation
4. Pain while seminal fluid is being ejaculated
5. Premature ejaculation or impotence
6. A chronic feeling that the bowels are filled up and there is difficulty in elimination
7. Any decrease in self-control over voiding, such as difficulty in beginning or stopping the stream or an inability to slow the stream

For any prostate difficulty, it is important to visit a physician or urologist (physician who specializes in disorders of the urinary or genitourinary systems) for a complete diagnosis. Any of these seven symptoms may suggest prostate disorder or may be symptomatic of another condition which your doctor can treat.

Researchers Peter P. Lamy and Mary Ellen Kitler, presenting a study made at Johns Hopkins University on physiologic and pathologic changes that occur in people as they grow older, state that many men take it for granted that enlargement of the prostate gland will occur when they get older. Reporting in the *Journal of the American Geriatric Society* (October 1971), they state:

"It is claimed that 30 percent of the male population will have some enlargement of the prostate at age 60 or above, that gross prostatic enlargement occurs in 30 to 50 percent of males over 60, and that there is a prostatic enlargement in 76 percent of males over 55."

### Pollen: Key to Prostate Health

Bee pollen as a means of keeping the prostate healthy was mentioned, for the first time in 1959, by a Swedish physician, Erik Ask-Upmark, M.D., of the University of Uppsala. Writing in *Grana Palynologica,* in an article called "On a New Treatment of Prostatitis," the doctor starts off by saying, "Prostatitis represents a relatively new pathologic entity. When I was studying medicine, one heard of its existence, but chiefly as a patho-anatomic curiosity. It was not, on the other hand, seen in the clinics, at any rate not in medical ones." The doctor was anxious to find out why prostate trouble is on the increase and what could be done about it.

Dr. Ask-Upmark tells of treating a patient who had prostate infection and suffered for five years; he was given a large dose of Chloromycetin (an antibiotic) but it offered no help. The patient then started to take bee pollen supplements on his own initiative. Dr. Ask-Upmark reports that the patient was examined for a period of two years while he was on the bee pollen program and that there were no symptoms. His prostatic disorder had healed or been cleared up. When the patient took a trip and left the supplements behind, there was some symptomatic recurrence. Apparently, pollen could heal the prostate for this man.

Says Dr. Ask-Upmark, "The patient took six tablets

a day of bee pollen extract. The improvement was like a miracle. He has had no trouble with his prostate."

The symptoms of prostatitis are described by Dr. Ask-Upmark:

"Prostatitis occurs both in an acute form and as a chronic disease, in which acute exacerbations [sharp] in the form of pain are highly characteristic.

"The local symptoms can most simply be described as those of cystitis, i.e., a continual urge to void and discomfort on urination. Prostatitis has, however, certain typical features. *Firstly*, the discomfort on urination consists far more of pain than of burning. *Secondly,* this pain is often referred to the tip of the penis, approximately as in the presence of an advanced vesical calculus [stone]. *Thirdly*, the patient may have a sensation of fullness in the rectum, which can reasonably be ascribed to bulging of the swollen prostate gland into it. This makes the patient try to relieve his discomfort by (unsuccessful) defecation. These local symptoms are accompanied, in the acute phase, by systemic disturbances in the form of fever."

With publication of Dr. Ask-Upmark's case history of the man who healed his symptoms by the use of bee pollen and nothing else, other doctors started to use bee pollen as a healer.

In 1962, Gosta Leander, M.D., a Swedish doctor, tested some 179 males who had problems of prostate infection. As reported in the *Swedish Medical Journal* (59 [1962]), he first started to give the patients "conservative treatment" of periodic massages that would help to remove wastes or substances that could be infectious. Then he set up a study as a double-blind test, using both pollen extract and placebos. Neither patients nor the doctors involved in the three-month study were aware (until the conclusion of the test) who was getting the real pollen and who was getting the dummy pills. Not even Dr. Leander knew which patients were getting the real pollen; he kept records by code number only.

Dr. Leander tells how he evaluated the study. "When an infection is in progress, the prostate and the vesicles have doughy consistency, they are tender when palpated and they contain a more or less pus-filled secretion.

"When therapy is successful, evacuation is improved and, consequently, the secretionary stasis (stoppage of normal flow of fluids) is eliminated. This can be easily confirmed by palpation. Concurrently, the secretion reverts to normal and this, too, is easily confirmed by direct microscopy."

Dr. Leander found that those patients who received pollen in their diet were healed better than those who did not. He says that 60 to 80 percent were better than those who were given conventional treatment only. Therefore, it seemed apparent that bee pollen could promote healing.

Another physician of Sweden, Gosta Jonsson, M.D. reporting in the *Swedish Medical Journal* (58:2487, nr36), tells of relieving five of his patients who suffered from prostate infections by giving them bee pollen over a period of a year's time. He also helped bring relief to another set of five patients who took bee pollen but not on a regular basis. Dr. Jonsson says, "Judging from observations made on ten patients who had been under observation for more than one year, the results are encouraging and warrant further trials with the bee pollen preparation. Uninterrupted treatment for a long period appears to be necessary if good results are to be expected."

Exactly what is the so-called miracle healing power of bee pollen, especially as related to prostate disorders? We may well look to its rich storehouse of nutrients—the same nutrients that have been taken out of processed foods. In particular, bee pollen contains magnesium, which is needed to nourish the prostate gland. Bee pollen is rich in those essential fatty acids needed to create prostaglandins or hormones which have an energizing activity upon the prostate. Bee pollen also contains zinc, which is needed for nourishment of the sex glands and the testicles.

A paper was presented by Arne Bolinder, Division of Food Chemistry, Royal Institute of Technology, Stockholm, on the subject of bee pollen. It was given at the meeting of the Swedish Association of Urologists on May 26, 1965, at the Karolinska Institute of Stockholm.

Dr. Bolinder studied the nutritive composition of bee pollen, and stated that the supplements "contain high contents of many nutrients of importance to the human body, i.e., essential amino acids and water-soluble vitamins.

". . . The content of nucleic acid derivatives is, quite probably, also rather high. Studies carried out to date of inorganic components have shown that zinc alone occurs in an amount which is unusually high for plant material."

## Correct Prostate Disorders with Bee Pollen

The very high zinc content of bee pollen may be a clue as to its value in healing the prostate gland. Zinc is found in just about all substances of reproduction in nature. Flowering plants, for example, are able to become fertilized and produce seeds because of pollination. Pollen is a prime source of zinc which the plants use to make seeds. Seeds themselves contain all the essential ingredients needed for sustaining new plant life. Seeds are prime sources of zinc. The reproductive organs of all animals, including man, are saturated with important zinc.

Scientists reported to the *Canadian Journal of Medical Sciences* (vol. 30, pp. 336-39) that zinc could be found in highly concentrated stores in the healthy prostate gland, and also in the sperm-nourishing seminal fluid secreted by the prostate.

Researchers reported to the *Journal of the American Medical Association* (April 11, 1959), that the prostate is high in zinc content, along with semen. "Sperm are richer in zinc than any human tissue studied, yet the testes are relatively poor in this element. From this observation alone, it would seem that zinc is related to spermatic physiology."

A deficiency in zinc may lead to changes in the size, structure and function of the prostate. Drs. Irving M. Bush, Alfred Zamm and their colleagues at Chicago's Cook County Hospital determine if the prostate is deficient in zinc by testing samples of semen. They find that seven out of ten men have low zinc levels while three out of ten are borderline. They have also found that they can produce increases in zinc levels in the semen and improve health of the prostate gland with proper supplementation. Bee pollen, a highly concentrated source of zinc, is important in boosting zinc levels of the prostate and the semen. The doctors say that increased zinc will also help heal the nonbacterial prostatitis. And . . . pollen has a high concentrate of zinc in its natural form, hence its use by doctors and scientists for treatment and rejuvenation of the prostate gland.

Research at Winnipeg (Canada) Hospital, decades ago, revealed that a zinc deficiency can render the prostate gland weak and vulnerable to cancer. Doctors at the hospital (*Cancer* 9, 1956: 721–26) showed that if a male had a 35 percent drop in zinc from normal levels, there was "a mild enlargement of the prostate gland." When there was a 38 percent drop in zinc, there was "chronic prostatitis." When zinc dropped by two-thirds, "the prostate gland developed into a cancerous infection."

In June 1976, at the annual convention of the American Medical Association, William Pories, M.D., a pioneer in zinc research, told the gathering of doctors that zinc was needed to give new life, to cause a proliferation of new cells and rejuvenation of tissues. Dr. Pories emphasized that a very tiny but powerful amount of zinc is found in enzymes which prompt the growth of tissues and organisms. So zinc is an all-important nutrient. Dr. Pories emphasized that a deficiency of zinc would cause growth retardation, delay the healing of wounds and specifically impair fertility.

While zinc is found in many foods such as organic or fertilized eggs (fertile hens' eggs are high in zinc because of the presence of the male sperm, while incubator eggs are low in zinc since they are artificially induced), pumpkin seeds, sunflower seeds, nuts, whole grains and leafy vegetables, *the most potent source of zinc is bee pollen!*

For a full year, G. W. Heise of the Magdeburg Academy of Medicine in Germany, treated nine patients with prostate disorder. All had symptoms such as difficulty in voiding, pain, urgency and frequency. Dr. Heise reported that all had clearly defined "difficulties during coitus." An examination showed they had white blood cells (leukocytes) in their ejaculates. The nine men had problems of very low libido as well as painful orgasm. Six of them were about to surrender to impotence. Dr. Heise began his treatment. The nine men were instructed in taking pollen regularly. Doses were individually prescribed. After a period of treatment, Dr. Heise found that *"all of the patients had responded with a definite improvement."*

The use of pollen had worked wonders of healing. Dr. Heise reports that their ejaculates showed them to be free of bacteria and leukocytes. "In all cases, this clearing up occurred after the nine men took one tablet of pollen, three times daily." The pollen also cleared up their disease-causing bacteria. All of the men now showed improved mental and physical health. Dr. Heise says:

"Cohabitation difficulties no longer occur. Pains radiating to the perineum and sacral region have disappeared. Micturition [urination] disturbances could no longer be observed . . .

"It would be a commendable advance if treatment

with this bee pollen preparation were to become incorporated into recommended therapeutic praxis [healing practice]."

So we can see that by adding pollen to the diet, its ingredients tend to bolster the vigor of the prostate gland so that it can fight infection and help clear up infectious bacteria. Apparently, the various nutrients in pollen can create this self-cleansing reaction. It is believed that discovered hormones in pollen are also beneficial to the prostate.

A group of scientists in Yugoslavia conducted tests with bee pollen at the University of Zagreb. As reported in *Experientia*, a Yugoslav scientific journal (1971), they found that pollen of the Scotch pine contains traces of estrogens, testosterone, epitestosterone and androsterone. All of these are hormones. While quantities are small, they are potent and believed to be of great value to the healing and maintenance of the prostate gland. They are also believed to promote an invigorating and strengthening effect upon the entire body.

Bee pollen is beneficial to the prostate gland even if there is little or no bacterial infection, but just a mild disorder. So reports L. J. Denis, M.D., a urologist in Antwerp, Belgium, in *Acta Urologica Belgica* (January 1966). Dr. Denis treated a group of men who had prostatitis but with no bacterial infection. These men were each given four tablets of bee pollen a day. Dr. Denis says:

"The mean age was 36. Slight urinary problems were present in each instance which was mainly the reason for their reference. These included frequency, urgency, hesitation, discomfort when urinating. None of them complained of urethral discharge. Three of them complained of loss of sexual desire and four had regular pain in one of the testicles, groin or perineum." Yet, the taking of four tablets a day, each, for a prescribed amount of time, gave them relief and they "no longer complained of the symptoms."

Bee pollen has a high concentrate of aspartic acid. This amino acid is used to treat chronic fatigue and sexual weakness. Bee pollen also contains steroid hormones as well as the gonadotropic hormone, spurring on the pituitary to release hormones that nourish the reproductive glands. Taking bee pollen which contains these ingredients can help correct disorders of the libido and offer a sexual boosting reaction.

As reported in *Prevention* (January 1975), a man had difficulties with his prostate.

"With the vitamins I was taking, I added bee pollen. My urologist had been suggesting a prostate gland removal but after a pyelogram X ray [picture of the kidney], he told me I had improved.

"He said there was still some enlargement of the prostate but not enough to cause any distress. He told me to see him again three months later.

"I believe that adding bee pollen to my other vitamins and changing to a more nutritious diet helped my prostate to start returning to normal. I still eat bee pollen. I am 70 years of age and walk at least three miles out in the air every day."

If it is true that a male is as young as his prostate,

then bee pollen may well be the elixir or ambrosia needed to keep his gland young and healthy. It is the all-natural way to boost body-mind health, through a pollen-nourished prostate gland.

# CHAPTER 9

## *LOOK YOUNGER WITH BEE POLLEN*

Your skin can become younger looking, less vulnerable to wrinkles, smoother and healthier with the use of bee pollen. Such is the discovery made by Lars-Erik Essen, M.D., of Hälsingborg, Sweden, who is considered a pioneer in the use of this rejuvenating food product. As a dermatologist, Dr. Essen treated many of his patients for acne. He developed a pollen lotion (currently in wide use throughout Sweden as well as other countries of Northern Europe) that could actually halt the spread of skin disease and also promote a smoothing down and easing of wrinkles and furrows.

Acne is traced to various causes: hormonal imbalance, nutritional deficiencies or infection. Pollen lotion reportedly is able to help halt the spread of acne and then enable the body to correct the errors so that self-healing then takes place. Dr. Essen says that pollen lotion suppressed the occurrence of new pustules (tiny, blisterlike spots) on the skin, then it nourished the skin and improved its general health.

Not only does pollen help clear up acne conditions in the young, says Dr. Essen, but it is also of special benefit in skin rejuvenation for older people. Says Dr. Essen: "Through transcutaneous nutrition, bee pollen has a profound biological effect. *It seems to prevent premature aging of the cells and stimulates the growth of new skin tissue. It offers effective protection against dehydration and injects new life into dry cells. It smooths away wrinkles and stimulates the life-giving blood supply to all skin cells.*"

Bee pollen is an important skin rejuvenator because it contains a high concentration of the nucleic acids, RNA and DNA. These substances penetrate the surface of the skin when a lotion containing bee pollen is applied, and they nourish the cells and tissues beneath. They act as a moisturizer for dry skin subject to wrinkling and premature aging, and also help smooth furrows and creases that cry out "old age."

Improve the look and feel of your skin (hair, too) with the use of bee pollen in all-natural beauty aids that you can prepare at home at a cost of just pennies. Here is an assortment of folk remedies that use bee pollen as an ingredient with other natural foods and help revitalize and rejuvenate your body and help you glow with youthful alertness.

SUGGESTION: At your local health store or pharmacy, obtain bee pollen in pellet form. Break open the pellet and let the tiny grains spill out onto a spoon for specific measurements. Or purchase free-flowing grains from the health store or pharmacy. Use the grains as soon after purchase as possible so they are fresh and potent.

### Facial Cleanser

Beat the yolk of an egg until it is light and frothy. Add ½ cup milk, ½ mashed, ripe, peeled avocado and 1 teaspoon bee pollen grains. A blender is handy here, but if you don't have one, beat the mixture with a fork until you have a thin cream or lotionlike consistency. Apply with squares of cotton as you would any other cleanser.

You may also use this deep cleaner *after* ordinary soap and water, if your skin is normal. It's a very pure method of keeping your complexion free of pollutants and grime which can interfere with normal skin function.

Since this formula is perishable, it is best to make it every other day and store in the refrigerator between uses.

### Spice Astringent

In a measuring cup, combine 2 tablespoons lemon juice, 1 tablespoon glycerin and 1 tablespoon 70 percent alcohol. Add 1 tablespoon bee pollen grains, then just enough distilled witch hazel to fill the cup to the 8-ounce level. Stir vigorously with a spoon. Refrigerate only until tingly cool. Then apply with your fingertips.

Let the astringent soak into your pores most of the day.

### Skin Pep Tonic

Combine 2 tablespoons buttermilk, 1 teaspoon bee pollen grains and 4 tablespoons tomato juice in a blender or hand-stir vigorously. Apply on your skin with cotton pads. Let remain up to 30 minutes, then splash off with cool water.

### Face Scrub

Peel and mash a ripe avocado (½ should be enough). Mix it with ½ cup yellow or white fine-grind cornmeal. Add 1 tablespoon bee pollen grains. Now, thoroughly wash your face in warm and then cold water. Next, rub this mixture into the trouble spots on your face. Continue rubbing for 10 minutes. Then remove with a damp washcloth and splash your face with cold water. The grains, combined with the other ingredients, help to slough off dead skin tissues, smooth out wrinkles and erase crease lines.

### Herb Rinse

To a cup of freshly boiled water, add ¼ cup fresh parsley, 1 teaspoon dried peppermint leaves, 1 teaspoon bee pollen grains. Let steep at least 30 minutes. Now strain through a cheesecloth. Pour into a clean glass bottle and use as an after-rinse, following your washing.

## Neck and Jawline Rejuvenator

Puree ½ avocado. Stir into it 1 tablespoon fresh wheat germ oil and 1 tablespoon bee pollen grains. You should now have a smooth cream. Rub this cream into your neck and jawline areas with firm strokes, going up and down and up and down. When most of the cream has been absorbed, remove the excess and leave on the residue for at least an hour or overnight. Use daily or nightly.

## Pore Tightener

In a clean bottle, combine 4 tablespoons rose water, ½ teaspoon spirits of camphor, 1 teaspoon bee pollen grains and 2 teaspoons alcohol (70 percent strength). Shake thoroughly until combined and keep in cool place. To use, apply with cotton pads over the entire skin area, rubbing into those sections which have large pores. Let remain overnight. Next morning, splash off with cool water.

## Facial Mask

Mix ½ mashed avocado, 1 tablespoon honey, ¼ cup whole milk and 2 tablespoons bee pollen grains. Either do it in a jar by hand or else blenderize the ingredients. They must all homogenize perfectly. (Having all ingredients at room temperature helps.) Now, clean your face and throat thoroughly. With your fingers, apply this mask to trouble spots on your skin, including your shoulders and back. Let remain for 30 minutes, then splash off with tepid water and a sponge or cloth. Follow with a brisk patting of ice water.

### Dry Skin Mask

Beat an egg yolk until it is light and frothy. Then add the mashed pulp of ½ avocado and 2 tablespoons bee pollen grains, blending them in thoroughly. Wash your face and throat before applying this mask. Now spread the mixture over your face and neck evenly; relax on a slant board or a bed for about 20 minutes. Remove with clear, tepid water and a facecloth, followed by a rinse of cold water or a milk skin lotion.

### Oily Skin Mask

Put the white of an egg, 1 teaspoon lemon juice, 2 teaspoons bee pollen grains and the mashed pulp of ½ avocado into a blender. In seconds, you should have a lovely green mixture. Or beat vigorously by hand. Wash your face and neck very thoroughly, then apply the mask evenly. Relax for 20 minutes; remove with tepid water and a facecloth. Follow with cold astringent.

### Skin Rejuvenator

In a small bowl or custard cup, mix 2 tablespoons instant, nonfat dry milk with 2 tablespoons water. Add 2 teaspoons bee pollen grains and continue mixing until you have a rather thick paste. To this add ¼ peeled, ripe avocado which has been well mashed (no lumps!).

Mix the ingredients together until you have a pale green cream. Apply this to your clean skin and leave on until you begin to feel your skin stiffen. Then add another layer. When that dries (about 10 minutes), remove the mask with tepid water and a cloth. Rinse well with clear water.

### Healthier Hair

Add a few drops of freshly squeezed lemon juice and bee pollen grains to your favorite shampoo. Then use as usual. Your hair will be left with a new, shiny and vibrant appearance.

### Softer Feet

Soak your feet in a mixture of comfortably hot water, 1 teaspoon bee pollen grains and the juice of 1 lemon. Just enjoy the soak until the water starts to cool. Then rinse off in warm water and dry carefully.

### Pollen Scrub

About once a week, your face should be given a good scrubbing to get rid of the dull, muddy look that comes from not quite removing all the dirt and excess oils that accumulate throughout the day. Here's how to prepare your pollen scrub: mix together the juice of 1 lemon and the white of 1 egg. Add 1 teaspoon bee pollen grains. Now add dry oatmeal gradually until you have a soft paste. Mix with a slight chopping motion, then allow to set a few minutes until the moisture is absorbed. Apply to your face, avoiding areas around the eyes. Rub in gently with a very tender scrubbing motion. Let dry about 10 minutes, then rinse off with clear, warm water.

### Ice Rub

To give your face a little pick-me-up on a hot day (or any day), fill an ice cube tray with equal parts strained lemon juice and water and 3 tablespoons bee pollen grains. Freeze. Whenever you want to refresh your face, remove one of the cubes and lightly rub over your face and neck. Rinse with cold water and pat dry. This leaves your face feeling as refreshed as if you'd splashed it in a mountain stream.

### Pollen Lotion

A good thing to keep in your refrigerator at all times is a bottle of pollen lotion. Mix it up in any quantity you like, using this formula: For every cup of strained lemon juice, add 1 teaspoon bee pollen grains and ½ cup water. Shake together. Keep it refrigerated. Use it for a facial, as a base for mixing with other cosmetics or as a splashing tonic to revive tired or aging skin.

### Pollen Youth Bath

Fill a tub with comfortably warm water. Add ½ cup bee pollen grains and a sliced fresh lemon. The lemon oils will release their sun-blessed fragrance and combine with the nectar-scented inhalation flavors of the grains to make you feel as if you are in a luxurious enchanted forest, bathing in an ambrosia-filled stream. Indulge yourself for 30 or even 60 minutes in this pollen youth bath, and emerge with the radiant glow of health and vitality.

## All-Purpose Cream

Blend together a peeled, very ripe banana, a peeled, ripe avocado and 2 teaspoons bee pollen grains. When thoroughly blended, you will have a cream that can be applied easily with your fingertips. Helps correct dryness, feelings of roughness and wrinkles. Use this all-purpose cream regularly. Leave it on up to 60 minutes, then rinse or splash off. Store the unused portion in a covered glass jar in your refrigerator but plan to use within 2 days.

## Salt Pollen Rubdown

This is a wonderful way to get satin-smooth skin all over your body. This prebath or preshower program is very invigorating. It can also be a great help in removing and healing blemishes on your shoulders and back. NOTE: It may be too strong for your delicate facial tissues, so test on a portion of your face as large as a thumbnail. If no irritation is felt, use gently on the rest of your face.

Mash ½ peeled avocado with ½ cup ordinary table salt and 2 tablespoons bee pollen grains. When thoroughly combined, rub the entire mixture all over your body, with particular emphasis on trouble spots. Use much friction. (Do it in your tub or shower.) Dead skin will sluff off in a miraculous way, especially on your feet, knees and elbows. When you think you've had enough, shower off and then bathe as usual.

## Easy Skin Cleanser

First prepare the almond meal. Toss blanched, skinless almonds into your blender and whizz until they are the consistency of grated Parmesan cheese.

Then make a paste out of 3 teaspoons almond meal, 3 teaspoons whole milk and 1 teaspoon bee pollen grains. Spread over your freshly washed and still moist skin. Let remain 20 minutes. Splash off with warm water, and final rinse will cool water.

## Pollen Soap Substitute

Mix together 1 egg yolk, 1 tablespoon glycerin, 1 teaspoon bee pollen grains. Gently pat onto your face. Let dry. Then splash off with warm water. Keep a supply in a closed jar in your refrigerator and always shake well before using. This is a skin-nourishing soap substitute for those who do not want an alkaline soap on their skin.

## Moisturizing Bath

Help replace lost moisture from your skin (cause of wrinkles and aging) by using this skin recipe. In a tub of warm water, add 2 tablespoons bee pollen grains, 2 teaspoons glycerin, 2 teaspoons pure peppermint extract. With your hand, swirl the water around so the ingredients blend together. Then soak yourself for 45 minutes. The warm water will open your skin pores and let the ingredients soak within to help moisturize the "reservoirs" lying directly beneath your skin surface. Smooths out entire body.

### Berry Rose Pollen Lotion

Press out the juice of 1 cup fresh ripe, cleaned strawberries through a sieve into a bowl. This should make about ½ cup rich red juice. To this, add ½ cup (4 ounces) rose water (available at health stores or pharmacies). Then add 2 teaspoons bee pollen grains. Stir. Chill before use (or else add an ice cube to the mixture before you pat it on your face). With fingertips, spread over your face. Let it remain for 20 minutes, then rinse with clear water. This lotion may be left on all night so the pollen can condition your skin while you sleep. The lotion will keep for about two days if well refrigerated.

### Night Body Oil

Combine 1 tablespoon each: sesame oil, light mineral oil, safflower oil, corn oil and bee pollen grains. Add 3 drops oil of bitter almonds (from herbal pharmacist) and shake together very thoroughly in a glass bottle. After your evening shower or bath (when your body pores are still open from the warm steam vapors), apply this night body oil onto your skin in a very light film. Rub gently deep into your skin. Then put on your nightclothes and have a good night's sleep. Next morning, shower or bathe with tepid water, and your skin should have a silky soft feeling. Repeat frequently for a younger skin that glows with youthful radiance.

## Dandruff Away Lotion

In a glass bottle, shake 1 cup white vinegar, 1 cup water, 2 tablespoons bee pollen grains. Dab this solution, using cotton pads, onto your scalp before shampooing. Rub it in well. When your entire scalp and hair have been covered, wash your hair with your favorite shampoo. Ingredients in the dandruff away lotion help loosen scalp debris and dandruff and will help cleanse your scalp and leave your hair looking and feeling squeaky clean.

## Dry Hair Pollen Treatment

In ½ cup mayonnaise (or mayonnaise-type salad dressing) stir 1 teaspoon bee pollen grains. Gently massage this mixture into your scalp and hair. Let it soak up to 45 minutes to have a natural penetrating reaction, rinse out under tepid water, then shampoo. This helps moisturize scalp cells and correct problems of dry hair. Repeat at least 3 times a week.

## Scalp Nourishing Tonic

Simmer 1 cup water. Into this add 1 tablespoon linseed oil and 1 teaspoon bee pollen grains. Puncture 1 vitamin A and 1 vitamin E capsule and squeeze the contents into the simmering water. Stir until ingredients are dissolved. Then cool mixture until comfortable to the touch but still warm. Apply to your scalp and hair. Soak your entire head in this mixture. Cover your head with a plastic shower cap to seal in body warmth and keep scalp pores open so this tonic can "feed" your hair follicles. After 30 minutes, remove cap and rinse your hair under tepid water. Shampoo as customary. Repeat 3 or more times per week. Nutrients in this scalp-nourishing tonic help feed your hair follicles and promote healthier growth.

# CHAPTER 10

## *HOW TO USE BEE POLLEN. WHEN? HOW MUCH?*

Bee pollen comes from many different floral sources. Just as with honey, bee pollen comes in all colors and tastes. Some may be a little sweet. Other pollen may have a tangy taste. But all bee pollen is a source of healthful energy and healing powers. Therefore, experiment with different varieties until you find the one you like. Or else use variations throughout the week so your body system can be rewarded with different potencies, different flavors. Health stores and pharmacies have all varieties of bee pollen available for your personal satisfaction.

For better assimilation, take pollen before eating. Take whatever amount is prescribed on the box or bottle, since each form and variety differs from every other. But always be consistent in your schedule—stick to it. Pollen appears to be better absorbed and more speedily assimilated when it is taken before a meal, so make this your rule of thumb.

Follow label directions on how much to use. Depending on your personal requirements, you may want more or less potent doses than indicated. If you feel you need more protective measures or if you want to build stronger immunity to the threat of illness, then increase the amount of pollen. When your health has been built up, take a maintenance dosage daily. Again, this is determined only by your individual needs and feelings. And again, read labels.

Here are some suggestions on how to take the bee pollen:

1. Take the prescribed number of tablets or capsules with a fresh fruit or vegetable juice, hot beverage or a glass of water
2. Sprinkle one teaspoonful of grains on any fruit or vegetable salad
3. Sprinkle the pollen grains into yogurt
4. Mix with honey, health jam or marmalade and spread atop whole-grain bread
5. Sprinkle pollen grains in fruit cocktails or on fruit salads or in a gelatin dessert
6. Add pollen grains to any beverage made with a juice extractor or blender
7. *Most important:* establish your pollen-taking program and stick to it daily.

As a miracle food from nature, bee pollen is being hailed by scientists and physicians from all corners of the world as a hope for total youth.

Bee pollen is the natural way to help heal and regenerate your body and mind so that you will respond with youthful vigor.

Bees, even without being mentioned in association with birds, are well up on the list of mankind's most important friends. One obvious reason, of course, is that they produce bee pollen, an accomplishment that deserves at least an "important friend" rating.

Then there is their ability to produce beeswax as well as honey, products that are very vital to your health and well-being.

Bees contribute to your well-being even more: they pollinate. A few other insects spread pollen as they visit blossoms, but the bee is the most efficient and the only dependable pollinator. A high percentage of the plant-derived food you eat comes from plants dependent on or benefited by insect pollination. Most of the livestock products you eat come from animals that once consumed insect-pollinated plants. So perhaps two-thirds of your diet comes from insect-pollinated crops.

Bee pollen is "the stuff of which life is made." Use it . . . and discover a new—and longer—life span.

## ANALYSIS OF BEE

### Vitamins
1. Provitamin A
2. B$_1$Thiamine
3. B$_2$Riboflavin
4. B$_3$Niacin
5. B$_6$Group
6. Panthothenic acid
7. Biotin
8. B$_{12}$ (cyanocobalamin)
9. Folic acid
10. Choline
11. Inositol
12. Vitamine C
13. Vitamin D
14. Vitamin E
15. Vitamin K
16. Rutin

### Minerals
1. Calcium
2. Phosphorus
3. Potassium
4. Sulphur
5. Sodium
6. Chlorine
7. Magnesium
8. Iron
9. Manganese
10. Copper
11. Iodine
12. Zinc
13. Silicon
14. Molybdenum
15. Boron
16. Titanium

### Others
1. Nucleic acids
2. Flavonoids
3. Phenolic acids
4. Tarpenes
5. Nucleosides
6. Auxins
7. Fructose
8. Glucose
9. Brassins
10. Gibberellins
11. Kinins
12. Vernine
13. Guanine
14. Xanthine
15. Hypoxalthine
16. Nuclein
17. Amines
18. Lecithin
19. Xanthophylls
20. Crocetin
21. Zeaxanthin
22. Lycopene
23. Hexodecanal
24. Alpha-amino-butyric-acid
25. Monoglycerides
26. Diglycerides
27. Triglycerides
28. Pentosans

# POLLEN CONTENT

### Enzymes, co-enzymes
1. Amylase
2. Diastase
3. Saccharase
4. Pectase
5. Phosphatase
6. Catalase
7. Disphorase
8. Cozymase
9. Cytochrome systems
10. Lactic dehydrogenase
11. Succinic dehydro-
    genase
12. 24 oxidoreductases
13. 21 transferases
14. 33 hydrolases
15. 11 lyases
16. 5 isomerases
17. Pepsin
18. Trypsin

### Proteins/amino acids
1. Isoleucine
2. Leucine
3. Lysine
4. Methionine
5. Phenylaline
6. Threonine
7. Tryptophan
8. Valine
9. Histidine
10. Arginine
11. Cystine
12. Tyrosine
13. Alanine
14. Aspartic acid
15. Glutamic acid
16. Hydroxyproline
17. Proline
18. Serine

# CLINICAL TREATMENT WITH POLLEN, OF PATIENTS WITH PSYCHICAL AFFECTIONS

R. LLOPIS PARET*
*Spain*

At the end of 1971 I started to use pollen as a thera-peutic in general psychiatry and the treatment of alco-holism. From the first moment the results were so satisfactory that I have introduced pollen into the medi-cation I systematically use in many patients. Unfortu-nately I never statistically recorded my results but I can say that by using pollen in a great number of cases for about three years, I obtained a good idea as to its use and possibilities, in the same way that a physician gains experience of the medicines he habitually admin-isters.

At the beginning, taking into account pollen composition and its possible application in my field, I selected three groups of patients suffering from the following affec-tions:

a) depressive syndromes
b) exhaustion or asthenia
c) alcoholism

## Depressive syndromes

Pollen alone cannot cure most cases of serious depres-sive syndromes. But it makes patients recover on small-er doses of drugs and in a shorter time than that neces-sary when no pollen is used.

* A doctor writing in *Apiacta*, a Spanish entomological journal.

But I consider more important another result obtained with depressive patients treated with pollen. All psychiatrists know that depressive persons are dependent on drugs. Patients recover or improve with drug administration, but when the dose is decreased or the antidepressive medicine is no longer administered, the depression usually reappears. Many a time, pollen has proved to be an efficient means of maintaining the patient in a normal state, without having to administer antidepressive drugs, not even in maintenance doses.

The most remarkable case I remember is that of a sixty-one-year-old patient, a waiter, married and having children; for seventeen years he had taken relatively high doses of Tofranil (between 100 and 150 mg daily, depending on periods), with various other tranquilizers. Starting with 2.5g pollen daily I could gradually reduce and finally discontinue the medication administered to this patient who, at present, takes only moderate or small doses of pollen from time to time; in one year and a half, no recurrence was recorded.

Not all cases are so spectacular but for all the depressions, pollen is an extremely useful adjuvant which I systematically use.

### Cases of exhaustion or asthenia

When psychiatrically examined, a great percentage of patients present a state of exhaustion, asthenia, melancholia, a decrease in the vital tonus, etc. The main causes of this syndrome lie in the present way of life: hard work and haste, constant environmental stress, bad emotional communication, etc.

In these cases pollen has proved to be an important energy-producing factor. After a few days of treatment, almost all patients show a subjective improvement. Their vital tonus increases, they have more energy to face environmental stress, their mood improves. This increase in the patient's vitality creates for him better conditions to successfully solve his psychological problems, if he has any, and provided they are not too complicated, or to start a course of psychotherapy. I must emphasize that I obtained good results in the psychotherapy of other types of patients with pollen as an adjuvant.

A special chapter could be dedicated to the cases where the decrease in the vital tonus is due to old age (including the so-called involution depressions or subdepressions), that is, to cases where the depressive syndrome is especially due to the general decrease of vital power which is characteristic of the biological involution and not to specific psychic or environmental factors. I very quickly obtained excellent results in such patients. However, in these cases, the treatment must be continued for a long time, in small doses (1g day). Of course, I sometimes also had to administer antidepressive drugs or tranquilizers but in most cases it was not necessary.

### Alcoholics

In my opinion, alcoholism is the field where pollen is most useful. As all people know, the chronic alcoholic lacks many vitamins and proteins for the remedy of which pollen is very efficient.

According to my experience pollen is most efficient in the abstinence syndrome which appears when the alcoholic stops drinking. Usually, this abstinence syndrome lasts for a short time—about one week on the average—but when using pollen (2-3g day) with small doses of Librium and an abundant water diet it can be reduced to 3 days or less, or it may not even appear.

I think this recommendation is important because in a great number of cases the abstinence syndrome is one of the factors which prevents the alcoholic from taking the decision to treat himself.

Therefore, the physician can promise the patient a short benign abstinence syndrome. The most serious complications of the alcoholic abstinence syndrome (i.e. delirium tremens and the Wieck alcoholic syndrome) did not appear in any of my patients treated with pollen and generally their recuperation was easier and quicker.

In conclusion, my experience shows that pollen is a very important therapeutic factor in psychiatry. During the past years, pollen has become one of the products I habitually use in my current practice.